高等院校数字化课程创新教材

供护理、助产及医学相关专业使用

护理英语（阅读分册）

English for Nursing (Reading)

主　编　罗晓冰　王炎峰

副主编　刘　杨

编　者　（按姓氏汉语拼音为序）

　　　　陈　爽　铁岭卫生职业学院

　　　　韩亚蕾　济南护理职业学院

　　　　李　静　泰山护理职业学院

　　　　刘　杨　济南护理职业学院

　　　　罗晓冰　承德护理职业学院

　　　　钱　超　泰山护理职业学院

　　　　宋洪玲　哈尔滨医科大学（大庆校区）

　　　　孙韵雪　广州卫生职业技术学院

　　　　王炎峰　重庆医药高等专科学校

　　　　余　可　重庆医药高等专科学校

　　　　张佳媛　哈尔滨医科大学（大庆校区）

　　　　赵　静　承德护理职业学院

科　学　出　版　社

北　京

U0230344

内 容 简 介

　　本教材依据护理岗位需要组织编写内容，内容编排以医院真实场景为主线，以临床护理工作为框架，以临床病例为导向，涉及基础护理、内科护理、外科护理、妇产科护理、儿科护理、精神科护理等护理专业理论及技能内容，以及医学影像技术、医学检验技术、用药护理、人际沟通技巧等相关知识。

　　本教材可供护理、助产及医学相关专业使用，亦可作为临床护理人员及拟出国工作的护理人员的参考读物。

图书在版编目（CIP）数据

护理英语（阅读分册）＝English for Nursing (Reading) / 罗晓冰，王炎峰主编. —北京：科学出版社，2019.8
高等院校数字化课程创新教材
ISBN 978-7-03-060309-8

Ⅰ. 护⋯　Ⅱ. ①罗⋯　②王⋯　Ⅲ. 护理学－英语－阅读教学－高等学校－教材　Ⅳ. R47

中国版本图书馆CIP数据核字（2019）第001086号

责任编辑：张立丽　辛　颖 / 责任校对：王萌萌
责任印制：赵　博 / 封面设计：金舵手世纪

科 学 出 版 社 出版
北京东黄城根北街 16 号
邮政编码：100717
http://www.sciencep.com
固安县铭成印刷有限公司 印刷
科学出版社发行　各地新华书店经销

*

2019 年 8 月第 一 版　开本：787×1092　1/16
2024 年 1 月第七次印刷　印张：12 1/4
字数：279 000

定价：45.00 元
（如有印装质量问题，我社负责调换）

前　　言

党的二十大报告指出："人民健康是民族昌盛和国家强盛的重要标志。把保障人民健康放在优先发展的战略位置，完善人民健康促进政策。"贯彻落实党的二十大决策部署，积极推动健康事业发展，离不开人才队伍建设。党的二十大报告指出："培养造就大批德才兼备的高素质人才，是国家和民族长远发展大计。"教材是教学内容的重要载体，是教学的重要依据、培养人才的重要保障。本次教材编写旨在贯彻党的二十大报告精神和党的教育方针，落实立德树人根本任务，坚持为党育人、为国育才。

随着医疗卫生和健康服务业的快速发展，护理专业国际化的发展趋势及国际人才市场的需求对护理及相关专业从业人员的英语应用能力提出了更高的要求。根据"职业教育即就业教育"的思想，本教材的编写团队本着以就业为导向、以能力为本位的观念，以满足岗位需要为目标，旨在培养适应现代社会需要的实用型护理专业人才。本教材体现护理专业特点，根据护理岗位需要组织内容，注重职业素养及职业能力培养，突出职业实用性和技能性。

《护理英语（阅读分册）》的内容编排以医院真实场景为主线，以临床护理工作为框架，培养学生护理英语的"应用能力"和"交际能力"。教材编写过程中，团队广泛收集分析国外原版护理英语及护理专业教材，密切结合医护英语水平考试（METS 二级和三级）大纲要求，分析参考美国 CGFNS 考试内容，为学生通过 METS 考试和未来出国培训打下坚实基础。本教材以日常的护理工作为题材，内容涉及基础护理、内科护理、外科护理、妇产科护理、儿科护理、精神科护理等学科的相关护理专业理论及技能，以及医学影像技术、医学检验技术、用药护理、人际沟通技巧等相关知识，让学生循序渐进地掌握护理专业英语知识，着重培养学生掌握相关术语及常用的表达方式，使其具备临床工作所需的较强的阅读能力，体现职业教育的技能型人才培养目标。

本册教材共有十八个单元，每个单元包括病例导入、健康教育对话、护理技术短篇阅读、疾病护理课文阅读、相关补充阅读以及医学术语六个部分。选材内容涉及病人入院、病人出院、用药管理、伤口护理、医学标本、医学影像、术前护理、术后护理及常见疾病护理等知识及常用护理技术。本教材可供护理、助产及医学相关专业使用，亦可作为临床护理人员及拟出国工作的护理人员的参考读物。

《护理英语（阅读分册）》的出版离不开主编、副主编和编者们的通力合作，各参编院校尤其是承德护理职业学院的大力支持，以及出版社的鼎力协作，在此，对各位编者表示衷心的感谢，向各参编院校及出版社表示诚挚的谢意。由于编写时间、水平有限，本书难免有不足之处，恳请各位专家及读者批评指正。

编　者
2023 年 8 月

Contents

Patient Admission

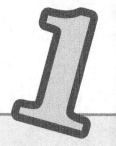

Learning Objectives:

1. *Taking a patient history*
2. *Writing a handover report*
3. *Discussing the nursing function of assessing vital signs*
4. *Providing information to clients about assessing vital signs*

Lead-In

Case Study

Mr. Frank, a 48-year-old man, had not been feeling well all day and at around 4 a.m., his wife awakened to see him slump to the floor, breathing with difficulty, and sweat was dripping. Alarmed when he told her of the pain in his chest, neck and arm, she called 120. At the emergency room, the patient's acute symptoms were relieved by the prompt action of the care team. Vital signs were stabilized, chest pain was relieved by nitroglycerin and the breathing was made easier by the increased oxygen flow. He was admitted to the coronary care unit (CCU).

Part 1 Dialogue

🎧 Taking a Patient History

Mr. Frank was admitted to the hospital because of a recent heart attack. Judy, the ward nurse, is filling out the Admission Form for him.

Judy:　　 Hello, it's Mr. Frank, isn't it?

Mr. Frank: Yes, that's right.

Judy:　　 My name is Judy. I'll be admitting you to the ward today. Would you mind if I check out some details first?

Mr. Frank: Not at all, dear. What do you want to know?

Judy:　　 First, I'd like to check your ID bracelet. Could you tell me your full name, please?

Mr. Frank: Yes, it's Chandler Frank and my date of birth is the seventh of July, 1959.

Judy:　　 Could you spell your first name for me, please?

Mr. Frank: OK. C-H-A-N-D-L-E-R.

Judy:	Thank you. And your date of birth is the seventh of July, 1959.
Mr. Frank:	That is correct.
Judy:	All right. Then, what brings you to the hospital today?
Mr. Frank:	Well, I had a heart attack last night and I'm here for some tests.
Judy:	OK. Next I'd like to ask you about your past medical history. Have you had any serious illness in the past?
Mr. Frank:	I've had lost my sleep for two years. It bothers me too much. I can't concentrate on anything.
Judy:	I'm sorry. It must be hard for you. Now what about the past surgical history of yours? Have you had any operations?
Mr. Frank:	I had my appendix out when I was twelve.
Judy:	Are you taking any medications these days?
Mr. Frank:	The doctor ordered some sleeping pills for me and I was told to bring them. Here they are.
Judy:	Very good. Let's see. It's diazepam. I'll write it down on the Admission Form. Do you have any allergies to medications?
Mr. Frank:	I'm allergic to penicillin.
Judy:	What about food allergies?
Mr. Frank:	No, not that I know of.
Judy:	All right. Now I need to know the name of your next of kin.
Mr. Frank:	It's my daughter. Rose Frank.
Judy:	Thanks. That's all for me. I'll get the admitting doctor to come and see you. Do you have any questions before I leave?
Mr. Frank:	No, thank you. Everything is all right.
Judy:	OK. If you need anything, please let me know.

🎧 Key Words

admission / ədˈmɪʃn / n. 接收入院

admit / ədˈmɪt / v. 接收入院

medical / ˈmedɪkl / adj. 医疗的；医药的

illness / ˈɪlnəs / n. 疾病

surgical / ˈsɜːdʒɪkl / adj. 外科的；手术的

operation / ˌɒpəˈreɪʃn / n. 手术

appendix / əˈpendɪks / n. 阑尾

diazepam / daɪˈæzəpæm / n. 安定

allergy / ˈælədʒi / n. 变态反应；过敏反应

allergic / əˈlɜːdʒɪk / adj. 过敏的

penicillin / ˌpenɪˈsɪlɪn / n. 青霉素

Useful Expressions

patient history   病史，病历

date of birth   出生日期

admission form   住院表格

next of kin   最近的亲属

Exercise

I Read the dialogue again and decide whether the following statements are right or wrong. If there is not enough information to answer "Right" or "Wrong", choose "Doesn't say".

1. The nurse is talking to Mr. Frank about heart attack. _____.

A. Right   B. Wrong   C. Doesn't say

2. Mr. Frank comes to the hospital because he lost his sleep. _____.

A. Right   B. Wrong   C. Doesn't say

3. The nurse tells Mr. Frank to bring the medication with him. _____.

A. Right   B. Wrong   C. Doesn't say

4. Mr. Frank is allergic to nothing but penicillin. _____.

A. Right   B. Wrong   C. Doesn't say

5. Mr. Frank puts his wife to be his next of kin. _____.

A. Right   B. Wrong   C. Doesn't say

II Discussion.

What information might you need to collect when taking a patient history?

Part 2 Short Passage

Handover Report

The handover report occurs two or three times a day on every type of nursing unit in all types of health care settings. At the end of each shift, nurses report information about their assigned clients to the nurses working on the next shift. The purpose of this report is to provide better continuity of care among nurses caring for a client. A client who sees different nurses performing care in the same manner, will likely trust caregivers more.

A handover report may be given orally in person, or during rounds at the client's bedside. Oral reports are given in conference room with staff from both shifts. Reports given in person or during rounds permit nurses to obtain immediate feedback when questions are raised about the client's care.

The nurse should use a systematic approach to provide a detailed description of client's progress during the shift.

a. Background information: Include client's name, sex, age, medical diagnosis, and brief medical history.

b. Assessment data: Provide objective observations and measurements made by the nurse during the shift. Describe client's condition and any recent changes. The oncoming nurses will use data as a baseline for comparison during the next shift.

c. Nursing diagnosis: Explain clearly the nursing diagnosis appropriate for client.

d. Interventions and evaluation: Describe treatments administered during shifts. Specify how interventions are uniquely given for this client. Explain client's response. Describe instructions given on teaching plan and client's ability to demonstrate learning.

e. Family information: Report on family visits. Explain if family members are included in care procedures.

f. Discharge plan: The client's progress in reaching discharge is reviewed on an ongoing basis during each handover report. The discharge plan identifies the interventions and outcomes needed to allow the client to have a smooth transition from the hospital to home.

g. Current priorities: Explain clearly the priorities to which the oncoming nurse must attend.

🎧 Key Words

handover / ˈhændəʊvə(r) / n. 交接
assigned / əˈsaɪnd / adj. 分配的
caregiver / ˈkeəgɪvə(r) / n. 看护者
feedback / ˈfiːdbæk / n. 反馈
systematic / ˌsɪstəˈmætɪk / adj. 系统的

diagnosis / ˌdaɪəgˈnəʊsɪs / n. 诊断
baseline / ˈbeɪslaɪn / n. 基线，底线
intervention / ˌɪntəˈvenʃn / n. 介入；干预
evaluation / ɪˌvæljuˈeɪʃn / n. 评估；诊断
priority / praɪˈɒrəti / n. 优先考虑的事

Useful Expressions

background information 背景信息
assessment data 评估资料

nursing diagnosis 护理诊断
discharge plan 出院计划

Exercise

I Choose the best answer to each question based on the text.

1. Which of the following descriptions about the nursing handover is NOT true? _____.

    A. Nurses can give a handover report at any time of the day

    B. The handover report is made by nurses from two different shifts

    C. One client may be cared for by more than one nurse

2. What does the word "feedback" in the second paragraph mean? _____.

    A. Comment   B. Response   C. Request

3. Why is it significant for nurse to provide objective observations and measurements? _____.

    A. Because the nurse from the next shift will know better about the client's condition

    B. Because it's a good way for the nurse to know the client's past history

    C. Because the medical staff will cooperate with each other in this way

4. After describing instructions given on teaching plan, the nurse should _____.

    A. initiate the treatment

    B. explain diagnosis

    C. make sure the client understand the teaching

5. The discharge plan is to _____.

    A. allow the client to be discharged from hospital as soon as possible

    B. allow the client to have a better transition from hospital to home

    C. allow the doctor to learn the client's condition well

Ⅱ Read the passage again and put the following extracts in the correct order.

☐ **A** Provide objective observations and measurements.

☐ **B** Explain nursing diagnosis.

☐ **C** Review discharge planning.

☐ **D** Explain priority.

☐ **E** Provide client's personal information.

☐ **F** Describe treatment and explain the client's response.

☐ **G** Report on family visits.

Part 3　Text

🎧 Vital Signs

Temperature, pulse, respirations, and blood pressure are known as vital signs. It is a basic nursing function in assessing the health status of an individual. These measurements are taken to help assess the general physical health of a person, give clues to possible diseases, and show progress toward recovery. Any difference between a patient's normal measurements and actual present vital signs is an indication for the nurse to give necessary medical care and initiate appropriate nursing therapies.

Under normal conditions, the normal human body temperature range is typically stated as 36.5-37.5 ℃ (97.7-99.5 ℉). Sites for measuring body temperature are oral, axillary (under the arm), rectal, and tympanic (in the ear). The common devices used to measure temperature are glass thermometers, electronic thermometers, and tympanic membrane thermometers. Many factors affect body temperature. These factors include age, gender, exertion, infection, and emotional state, etc. A person with an increased body temperature is referred to as febrile. On the other hand, a body temperature below the lower limit of normal is called hypothermia.

The pulse rate normally corresponds to the same rate at which the heart is beating. The rate and rhythm of the pulse may be assessed by compressing an artery against an underlying bone with the tip of the fingers. The heart rate can also be measured by listening to the heart beat by auscultation, traditionally using a stethoscope and counting it for a minute. The radial pulse is commonly measured using three fingers. An adult has tachycardia when the pulse rate is 100 to 180 beats per minute. When it falls below 60 beats, it is called bradycardia.

The movement of breathing involves the act of breathing in (inspiration) and breathing out (expiration). Generally speaking, healthy adults breathe about 16 to 20 times each minute. The nurse should aware that the unnoticed assessment of respirations immediately after the pulse assessment may prevent patient from conscious attempt to control breathing. If rhythm is regular, count number of respirations in 30 seconds and multiply by 2. In infant or young child, count for full minute. If adult has irregular rhythm or abnormally slow or fast rate, count for 1 full minute. Tachypnoea is indicated by a rate greater than 20 breaths per minute. Bradypnoea is abnormally slow breathing less than 16 breaths per minute.

Blood pressure is the force exerted by the blood against the vessel walls. It is usually expressed in terms of the systolic pressure (maximum during one heart beat) over diastolic pressure (minimum in between two heart beats) and is measured in millimetres of mercury (mmHg). Normal systolic blood pressure is 90 to 140 mmHg, and the normal diastolic blood pressure is 60 to 90 mmHg. Sphygmomanometer is used to measure blood pressure. It consists of a cuff, a manometer, and a stethoscope. Hypertension, also known as high blood pressure, is present if the resting blood pressure is persistently at or above 140/90 mmHg. Hypotension is blood pressure below 90/60 mmHg.

🎧 Key Words

axillary / ˈæksɪlərɪ / adj. 腋窝的
rectal / ˈrektəl / adj. 直肠的
tympanic / tɪmˈpænɪk / adj. 鼓膜的，鼓室的
thermometer / θəˈmɒmɪtə(r) / n. 体温计
febrile / ˈfiːbraɪl / adj. 发热的
hypothermia / ˌhaɪpəˈθɜːmɪə / n. 体温过低
auscultation / ˌɔːskəlˈteɪʃn / n. 听诊（法）

stethoscope / ˈsteθəskəʊp / n. 听诊器
tachycardia / ˌtækɪˈkɑːdɪə / n. 心动过速
bradycardia / ˌbrædɪˈkɑːdɪə / n. 心动过缓
tachypnoea / ˌtækɪpˈniːə / n. 呼吸急促
bradypnoea / ˌbrædɪpˈniːə / n. 呼吸过慢
hypertension / ˌhaɪpəˈtenʃn / n. 高血压
hypotension / ˌhaɪpəʊˈtenʃn / n. 低血压

Useful Expressions

vital signs   生命体征
tympanic membrane thermometer   耳温体温计
pulse rate   脉率

radial pulse   桡动脉脉搏
systolic pressure   收缩压
diastolic pressure   舒张压

Exercise

I **Choose the best answer to each question based on the text.**

1. According to the passage, which statement is true in assessing the vital signs?_____.

    A. The vital signs are the only clues to diseases

    B. The vital signs show if the patient's condition is better or worse

    C. The vital signs cannot help nurse give appropriate medical care

2. Which of the following is NOT mentioned as sites for measuring body temperature? _____.

A. Mouth   B. Rectum   C. Head

3. What can influence the body temperature? _____.

A. Food   B. Weather   C. Disease

4. Which of the following statements is true according to the text? _____.

A. Before counting number of the respirations, the nurse should tell the patient

B. It's better to assess the respirations without the notice of the patient

C. The nurse should ask the patient to control the breath when counting number of respirations

5. Which description is true about blood pressure? _____.

A. Normal systolic blood pressure is 60 to 90 mmHg

B. Normal diastolic blood pressure is 90 to 140 mmHg

C. One may suffer from hypertension when his/her blood pressure reaches 140/90 mmHg

II Match each medical term in Column A with its explanation in Column B.

Column A	Column B
_____	1. febrile	a. high blood pressure
_____	2. hypothermia	b. rapid breathing
_____	3. tachypnoea	c. subnormal body temperature
_____	4. bradycardia	d. abnormally slow heartbeat
_____	5. hypertension	e. characterized by fever

III Find words or terms in the article to match the following definitions.

1. listening to sounds within the body (usually with a stethoscope)   _____

2. abnormally rapid heartbeat (over 100 beats per minute)   _____

3. measuring instrument for measuring temperature   _____

4. a pressure gauge for measuring blood pressure   _____

IV Critical thinking.

According to the case at the beginning of this unit, what are nursing diagnoses and nursing interventions for the patient?

1. Nursing diagnoses

- Pain (acute) related to myocardial ischemia
- Anxiety related to pain, fear of death, and hospital environment
- Activity intolerance related to decreased cardiac output

2. Nursing interventions

On admission the patient is immediately placed on bed rest with a cardiac monitor and oxygen via nasal cannula or face mask. A series of ECGs is begun to establish the site of infarction or the presence of dysrhythmias. An intravenous line is established to provide the administration of medications. A low-cholesterol, salt-restricted diet is recommended. The patient is instructed to tell the nurse if any chest pain or shortness of breath occurs.

Part 4 Supplementary Reading

🎧 Nursing Assessment

Nursing assessment is the systematic and continuous collection, confirmation, and communication of client data; these data reflect how health functioning is enhanced by health promotion or compromised by illness. A database includes all the relevant client information collected by the nurse and other health care professionals; as such, it enables a comprehensive and effective plan of care to be designed and implemented for the client. The collection of client data is a vital step in the nursing progress because the remaining steps depend on complete, accurate, factual, and relevant data.

During the assessment step of the nursing progress, the nurse establishes the database by interviewing the client to obtain a nursing history; the nurse may also perform a nursing examination to collect data. Other sources of client information used by the nurse include the client's support people, the client record, the client's health care professionals, and nursing and other health care literature. After the nurse has established the database, data about the client are collected continuously because the client's health status can change quickly. All pertinent data are recorded and, when appropriate, verbally communicated to the responsible person, so that the data can best benefit the client.

There are two types of data—objective and subjective. Objective data are information perceived by the sense, and data observed by one person can be verified by another person observing the same client. Examples of objective data are an elevated temperature reading, skin that is moist, and refusal to look at or eat food. Subjective data are information perceived only by the affected person; these data cannot be perceived or verified by another person. Examples of subjective data are feeling nervous, nauseous, or chilly and experiencing pain.

Common methods used in the collection of data in nursing include observation, interview, and physical assessment. Observation is the conscious and deliberate use of the five senses to gather data. Interview is a planned communication. During the assessment step of the nursing progress, the nurse interviews the client to obtain a nursing history. Physical assessment is the examination of the client for objective data that may better define the client's condition and help the nurse in planning care.

Exercise

Choose the best answer to each question based on the text.

1. What does the word "database" mean in the first paragraph? _____.

    A. Collection of information

    B. Health promotion

    C. Effective plan

2. From whom can the nurse get the client's information? _____.

    A. The client's roommate   B. The client's friend

    C. The client's caregiver

3. Which of the following is NOT objective data? _____.

    A. Headache   B. Fever   C. Weight loss

4. Which of the following is subjective data? _____.

    A. Chest pain   B. Irregular breathing   C. High blood pressure

5. Which of the following methods is mentioned in the passage about collecting data? _____.

    A. Surgery   B. Planning   C. Observation

Part 5 Nursing Diagnosis

1. Altered Nutrition: More Than Body Requirements	营养失调：高于机体需要量
2. Altered Nutrition: Less Than Body Requirements	营养失调：低于机体需要量
3. Risk for Infection	有感染的危险
4. Risk for Altered Body Temperature	有体温改变的危险
5. Ineffective Thermoregulation	体温调节无效
6. Bowel Incontinence	大便失禁
7. Altered Urinary Elimination	排尿异常
8. Functional Incontinence	功能性尿失禁
9. Total Incontinence	完全性尿失禁
10. Urinary Retention	尿潴留
11. Altered Tissue Perfusion	组织灌注量改变
12. Fluid Volume Excess	体液过多
13. Fluid Volume Deficit	体液不足
14. Risk for Fluid Volume Deficit	有体液不足的危险
15. Decreased Cardiac Output	心排血量减少
16. Impaired Gas Exchange	气体交换受损
17. Ineffective Airway Clearance	清理呼吸道无效
18. Risk for Injury	有受伤的危险
19. Risk for Suffocation	有窒息的危险
20. Risk for Trauma	有外伤的危险
21. Risk for Aspiration	有误吸的危险

（赵　静）

Patient Discharge

Learning Objectives:

1. *Discussing patient confidentiality with clients or staff members*
2. *Referring a patient*
3. *Describing discharge planning in providing continuity of care*
4. *Planning a discharge for patient*

Lead-In

Case Study

William was a 58-year-old married man with a diagnosis of cerebrovascular accident (stroke) with left hemiparesis (weakness). He had difficulty communicating verbally and had a history of hypertension for 10 years. He was to be discharged from hospital in 3 days. He would be going home with four new medications, an indwelling urinary catheter, and a feeding tube. His wife did not believe she could manage care of the feeding tube and the catheter. She also needed instruction in the new medication and diet. How would the nurse coordinate this discharge plan?

Part 1 Dialogue

🎧 Confidentiality

Mary and Ryan, the ward nurses, are talking to the head nurse Kelly about patient confidentiality.

Kelly: Now, we're up to Mr. Conner in bed number 3 who was brought to hospital yesterday after taking an overdose of aspirin. I'm in charge of him. He's been quite settled after the treatment, but he seemed unstable mentally. He doesn't feel like talking for most of the time.

Mary: Yeah.

Ryan: Actually, I've just received a call from Mrs. Conner and she asked about her husband's present condition.

Mary: I don't think we're supposed to tell the family anything about the patient's diagnosis and treatment.

Ryan: I know. I remember there is confidentiality we've been taught back at school. That's why I didn't say anything to Mrs. Conner.

Mary: Yeah, right, the patient confidentiality. But I'm not quite sure about some of the rules. For example, what information do we need to keep confidential?

Kelly: Patients have a right to confidentiality. The law protects information about patients that is gathered by examination, observation, or treatment. Nurses are legally and ethically obligated to keep information about patients' illnesses and treatments confidential.

Mary: I understand the law protects the patients' privacy, but I just don't know how to respond properly when the family members ask about the patients health status.

Kelly: We can share the information with the next of kin only with the patients' permission. But we'd better tell them face to face, because we can't make sure whether he is a real family through phone or Internet.

Mary: I see what you mean.

Ryan: What about other medical staff?

Kelly: Most information is only passed to people involved in the health care. For example, the pharmacist who is responsible for giving drugs, or a radiologist reporting on X-rays. On some occasions, it may be necessary to pass information to another hospital if you need to make a referral for special treatment.

Ryan: And we should indicate with whom the information the patients give will be shared.

Kelly: Exactly. One more thing, try not to discuss the patients' illness in public places, such as the hall or the lift. And only provide the information to the relevant treatment team.

🎧 Key Words

confidentiality / ˌkɒnfɪˌdenʃiˈæləti / *n.* 机密性
overdose / ˈəʊvədəʊs / *n.* （用药）过量
aspirin / ˈæsprɪn / *n.* 阿司匹林
treatment / ˈtriːtmənt / *n.* 治疗
observation / ˌɒbzəˈveɪʃn / *n.* 观察

pharmacist / ˈfɑːməsɪst / *n.* 药剂师
radiologist / ˌreɪdiˈɒlədʒɪst / *n.* 放射科医生
X-ray / ˈeks reɪ / *n.* X光照片
referral / rɪˈfɜːrəl / *n.* 移交，送交

Useful Expressions

be in charge of   负责……
be obligated to   有责任去做

health status   健康状态
make a referral   转诊病人

Exercise

1 Read the dialogue again and decide whether the following statements are right or wrong. If there is not enough information to answer "Right" or "Wrong", choose "Doesn't say".

1. The nurses are talking about Mr. Conner's present condition. _____.

   A. Right   B. Wrong   C. Doesn't say

2. Ryan didn't tell Mrs. Conner about her husband's condition because of confidentiality. _____.

A. Right   B. Wrong   C. Doesn't say

3. Family members and close friends are free to know about patients' health status. _____.

A. Right   B. Wrong   C. Doesn't say

4. Medical staff involved in patients' health care have access to patients' records. _____.

A. Right   B. Wrong   C. Doesn't say

5. Nurses can discuss patients' illness in the doctor's office. _____.

A. Right   B. Wrong   C. Doesn't say

▌▌ Discussion.

Why is it important for patients to know that their personal information is kept confidential and in a safe place?

Part 2 Short Passage

🎧 Referring a Patient

Clients are referred to new agencies in order to receive different forms of therapy, to have care continued closer to home, and to have care continued when financial resources prohibit receiving care in the current facility. When clients are referred, many aspects of nursing care should continue as before. However, there will be changes if the medical plan of treatment is revised or if the agency's policies and procedures differ from those of the previous institution. The client expects care to continue as smoothly as possible without interruptions in therapy that may hinder progress toward recovery.

Because members of the two nursing staffs have minimal opportunity to communicate, the client's plan of care must be documented thoroughly in the medical record and on the referring form. It is important for members of receiving staff to have a clear understanding of the client's progress and current status. Telephone reports are often given between referring physicians. Primary nurses should take an active role in being sure the client's plan of care is clearly communicated either verbally or in written form.

Special equipments needed in support of client during transport are wheelchair or stretcher, oxygen tank or tubing, IV pole and cardiac monitor. The procedures of referral are recommended as:

1. Explain to client and family reasons for referral, when it is to occur, and what procedures are to be planned.

2. Make sure documentation in client's record is complete and accurate.

3. Obtain from client release form giving permission to have a copy of medical record made for receiving agency.

4. Complete nursing care referring form according to agency policy.

5. Gather client's personal care item, clothing, and valuables. Secure in suitcase or container.

6. Anticipate problems client may develop just before or during referral. Perform necessary

nursing therapies.

  7. Assist in referring client to stretcher or wheelchair using proper body mechanics.

  8. Perform final assessment of client's physical stability, that is, check vital signs, check for clear airway, inspect patency of intravenous lines, and note client's level of consciousness.

  9. Accompany client to transport vehicle.

  10. Call receiving agency and notify them of impending referral and client's status.

🎧 Key Words

refer / rɪ'fɜ:(r) / *vt.* 把……送往

therapy / 'θerəpi / *n.* 疗法，治疗

recovery / rɪ'kʌvəri / *n.* 恢复

physician / fɪ'zɪʃn / *n.* 内科医生

wheelchair / 'wi:ltʃeə(r) / *n.* 轮椅

stretcher / 'stretʃə(r) / *n.* 担架

stability / stə'bɪləti / *n.* 稳定（性）

airway / 'eəweɪ / *n.* （肺的）气道

intravenous / ˌɪntrə'vi:nəs / *adj.* 静脉注入的

consciousness / 'kɒnʃəsnəs / *n.* 意识

Useful Expressions

plan of care 护理计划

referring form 转诊单

oxygen tank 氧气瓶

patency of intravenous lines 静脉导管通畅性

Exercise

I **Choose the best answer to each question based on the text.**

1. The purpose of referring clients is NOT to help the clients _____.

  A. get back to work as soon as possible

  B. receive a continuous care from some place closer to home

  C. save medical expense

2. The nursing care of the referred client should remain the same except that _____.

  A. the client asks for a change

  B. the medical plan of treatment is revised

  C. the agency's policy is the same as the previous institution

3. Which of the following statements is NOT true according to the passage? _____.

  A. The receiving nurse should be responsible for the client's stable transition

  B. The client's plan of care should be recorded in detail in the medical record and on the referring form

  C. Medical staff can communicate with each other through telephone

4. After finishing the nursing care referring form, the nurse should _____.

  A. get permission to have a copy of medical record made for receiving agency

  B. gather client's personal care item, clothing, and valuables

  C. perform necessary nursing therapies

5. Which of the following responsibilities is correct concerning referring a patient? _____.

    A. Check if the client's IV is running properly

    B. Make sure the client has taken all the necessary belongings

    C. Both A and B

Ⅱ Read the passage again and put the following extracts in the correct order.

    ☐ **A** Inform the client of the time and procedure of referral.

    ☐ **B** Made a copy of the client's medical record for the receiving agency.

    ☐ **C** Complete the nursing care referring form.

    ☐ **D** Make sure the client has got all personal items with him/her.

    ☐ **E** Help client transport.

    ☐ **F** Perform final assessment of client's physical stability.

    ☐ **G** Call receiving agency and notify of the client's status.

Part 3 Text

🎧 Discharge Planning

Discharge planning is a systematic process of preparing the client to leave the health care agency and for maintaining continuity of care. The key to successful discharge planning is an exchange of information among the client, the caregivers, and those responsible for care both while the client is in the institution and after the client returns home. The coordination of care is usually the nurse's responsibility, but some hospitals have a nurse whose primary responsibility is to make the discharge planning.

Planning the discharge actually begins on admission, when information about the client is collected and documented. It is actually the same as the nursing process, by which a multidisciplinary team anticipates and plans for the needs of a client and family after discharge from a health care facility. Effective discharge planning also guarantees continuity of care in the least stressful manner. Discharge planning must:

- Be coordinated
- Be interdisciplinary
- Be initiated as early as possible
- Be carefully planned
- Involve the client, family, or significant others who are caregivers

With early discharge, clients often are still acutely ill when they go home, and many require complicated treatment and care by family members. It is no longer unusual for family members to change sterile dressings, monitor intravenous medications, give complete physical care, and prepare special diets. If they are unprepared for these interventions, the client may have an deterioration of the illness or experience complications that would require readmission to the hospital. The nurse must ensure that family members are taught the necessary knowledge and skills.

Initiation of the process involves identifying clients who need discharge planning. All clients need this service, but certain clients are at higher risk for specific needs and services. The nurse who conducts the initial nursing assessment is in the best position to determine these special needs. When assessing the client for discharge, the family is included as the unit of care. The client and family must be actively involved in the discharge process if the transition from hospital to home is to be effective. Nursing diagnoses, based on the discharge planning assessment, are developed to recognize the needs of both the client and the family. Information about medications, diet, procedures and treatments, referrals, and health promotion activities may be included in the teaching plan for discharge. All teaching should be documented in the nurse's notes and the discharge summary. Written instructions are given to the client. The client and caregiver must have exposure to and practice with the equipment they will be using at home. Evaluation of the discharge plan is crucial in making the discharge planning process work. Further evaluation is usually conducted a few weeks after the client has been home. It may be carried out by way of a telephone call, a questionnaire, or a home visit.

🎧 Key Words

discharge / dɪs'tʃɑːdʒ / n. 获准离开，出院
continuity / ˌkɒntɪ'njuːəti / n. 连续性
institution / ˌɪnstɪ'tjuːʃn / n. 机构
coordination / kəʊˌɔːdɪ'neɪʃn / n. 协调
multidisciplinary / ˌmʌltidɪsə'plɪnəri / adj. 多学科的
interdisciplinary / ˌɪntədɪsə'plɪnəri / adj. 跨学科的

acutely / ə'kjuːtli / adv. 急性地；剧烈地
sterile / 'steraɪl / adj. 无菌的
deterioration / dɪˌtɪəriə'reɪʃn / n. 恶化
complication / ˌkɒmplɪ'keɪʃn / n. 并发症
questionnaire / ˌkwestʃə'neə(r) / n. 调查问卷

Useful Expressions

health care agency   医疗机构
health care facility   医疗机构；医疗设施
nursing diagnosis   护理诊断

change dressings   换药
monitor intravenous medications   监护静脉给药

Exercise

I Choose the best answer to each question based on the text.

1. Which of the following statements is true according to the passage? _____.

   A. Discharge planning is to prepare a systematic care for the client during his/her stay in hospital

   B. On the day of discharge, the nurse starts to make the discharge plan for the client

   C. The discharge planning team includes the client, the caregivers, and those responsible for the care

2. Effective discharge planning is to ensure the _____ of care.

    A. quickness   B. honesty   C. continuity

3. Successful discharge planning should include the following characteristics except for being _____.

    A. cooperated   B. carefully planned   C. early initiated

4. What are the necessary knowledge and skills that the nurse should teach the family members?

    _____.

    A. How to start an IV fluid for the client

    B. How to make special meals for the client

    C. How to cope with complications

5. Which of the following statements is NOT true concerning discharge planning? _____.

    A. The family will determine what special service the client needs

    B. Nursing diagnoses recognize the needs of both client and family

    C. Evaluation can be carried out by a telephone call or a home visit

II Match each medical term in Column A with its explanation in Column B.

Column A		Column B
_____	1. sterile	a. leaving hospital with permission
_____	2. continuity	b. judging or assessing a person's condition
_____	3. deterioration	c. a stable condition without any interruption
_____	4. discharge	d. process of changing to an inferior state
_____	5. evaluation	e. free from bacteria

III Find words or terms in the article to match the following definitions.

1. a person who helps identifying, preventing or treating illness or disability _____

2. new development of an illness, that makes treatment more difficult _____

3. medical procedures or applications that are intended to relieve illness _____

4. the treating of illness by medical means _____

IV Critical thinking.

    According to the case at the beginning of this unit, what are nursing diagnoses and discharge planning made for the patient?

1. Nursing diagnoses

    • Altered physical mobility related to hemiparesis

    • Risk for injury related to impaired mobility

    • Impaired verbal communication related to dysarthria

2. Discharge planning

    Occupational therapist and speech and language therapist need to evaluate William's ability to perform activities of daily living and communication. The nutritionist needs to counsel his family on low-salt diet. Teaching plan for medication and treatment is necessary. His wife must learn about the urinary catheter and feeding tube before discharge. Making a referral to home health agency and continue physical therapy and nursing care. Transportation should be arranged at this time.

Part 4 Supplementary Reading

🎧 Nursing Planning

After the nurse collects and interprets client data, identifies client strengths and health problems, and prioritises nursing diagnoses, it is time to plan for nursing action. During the planning step of the nursing process, the nurse works with the client and family to identify client goal, that, if achieved, prevent, reduce, or eliminate the problems specialized in the nursing diagnoses, and identify the nursing interventions that are most likely to assist the client in achieving these goals.

The primary purpose of the planning step of the nursing process is to design a plan of care for and with the client that, once implemented, results in the prevention, reduction, or resolution of client health problems. A comprehensive plan of care specifies any routine nursing assistance the client requires to meet basic human needs (eg., assistance with hygiene or nutrition) and describes appropriate nursing responsibilities for fulfilling the medical plan of care. For example, physicians may delegate a surgical client to nurses for the redressing of the surgical incision, the administration of prescribed medications and intravenous therapy, and responsibility for scheduling laboratory studies. Nurses design plans of care that incorporate their independent and collaborative responsibilities. Because nursing is concerned with the client's responses to health and illness, the plan of care is supportive of nursing's broad aims—to promote wellness, prevent disease and illness, promote recovery, and facilitate coping with altered functioning.

Before developing or modifying the plan of care, it is helpful to review the prioritised list of nursing diagnoses to determine if they are correctly ranked as high priority (greatest threat to client's well-being), medium priority, and low priority (not specially related to current illness and prognosis). When planning for nursing care for each day, it is helpful to consider the following.

1. Have changes in the client's health status influenced what are considered the priority nursing diagnoses? For example, when a routine home visit of an older adult reveals evidence of possible elder abuse, a new set of priorities for care is needed.

2. Have changes in the way the client is responding to health and illness or the plan of care affected those nursing diagnoses that can be realistically addressed? For example, the nurse may have identified ineffective individual coping as a high-priority diagnosis for the client who has learned of the medical diagnosis, and planned to initiate counseling. But if the client adamantly

requests to be left alone for a day to think things through, the nurse has to modify priorities of care for that day.

3. Are there relationships between diagnoses that require that one be worked on before another can be resolved?

4. Can several client problems be dealt with together?

Exercise

Choose the best answer to each question based on the text.

1. Nursing planning is to _____.

    A. collect and interpret client data

    B. select the best interventions that help the client achieve goals

    C. specify nursing diagnoses

2. What is the purpose of nursing planning? _____.

    A. It identifies the current and future client care needs

    B. It designs a plan of care that helps with the client's health problems

    C. It specifies any basic human needs that the client requires

3. What is the correct order when the nurse determines the prioritised list? _____.

    A. High priority, medium priority, low priority

    B. Low priority, medium priority, high priority

    C. High priority, low priority, medium priority

4. Who should the nurse consider first when deciding the plan of care? _____.

    A. A client who is having a severe headache

    B. A client who is losing a lot of blood

    C. A client who is suffering from mild heart attack

5. Whose responses are the most important to be considered? _____.

    A. The nurse's   B. The client's   C. The doctor's

Part 5 Nursing Diagnosis

1. Impaired Tissue Integrity   组织完整性受损

2. Altered Oral Mucous Membrane   口腔黏膜改变

3. Impaired Skin Integrity   皮肤完整性受损

4. Risk for Impaired Skin Integrity   有皮肤完整性受损的危险

5. Decreased Adaptive Capacity Intracranial   调节颅内压能力下降

6. Risk for Deficient Fluid Volume   有体液不足的危险

7. Impaired Verbal Communication   语言沟通障碍

8. Impaired Physical Mobility   躯体移动障碍

9. Activity Intolerance　　　　　　　　　　活动无耐力，活动耐受力缺乏

10. Sleep Pattern Disturbance　　　　　　　睡眠状态紊乱

11. Feeding Self-Care Deficit　　　　　　　进食自理缺陷

12. Impaired Swallowing　　　　　　　　　吞咽障碍

13. Ineffective Breast Feeding　　　　　　　母乳喂养无效

14. Bathing/Hygiene Self-Care Deficit　　　　沐浴 / 卫生自理缺陷

15. Toileting Self-Care Deficit　　　　　　　如厕自理缺陷

16. Altered Growth and Development　　　　生长发育改变

17. Disorganized Infant Behaviour　　　　　婴幼儿行为紊乱

18. Impaired Memory　　　　　　　　　　记忆障碍

19. Risk for Self-Mutilation　　　　　　　　有自残的危险

20. Post-Trauma Response　　　　　　　　创伤后反应

（赵　静）

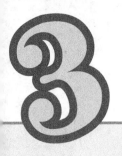 **Medication Administration**

Learning Objectives:

1. *Discussing the "five rights" of medication administration*
2. *Describing the intramuscular injection*
3. *Defining and classifying the routes of medication administration*
4. *Explaining the importance of skin allergy test*

Lead-In

Case Study

Mrs. Lenning was 78 years old who had been admitted for the investigation of cardiac problems. The ward nurse Anna and Paula were doing the medication assessment against the prescription chart. When they followed the "five rights" of medication administration for patient safety, they found some errors on the prescription chart. Mrs. Lenning was ordered Lasix and the doctor hadn't noted down the route and dose of medication. There was a problem with the frequency and time of administration as well.

Part 1 Dialogue

🎧 Discussing the "Five Rights"

Paula, a student nurse, is doing a medication assessment with Anna, a registered nurse.

Anna: Paula, are you ready to go through this medication assessment?

Paula: Yeah.

Anna: First, let's review. What are the "five rights"?

Paula: They are the right drug, the right patient, the right dose, the right route and the right time.

Anna: That's right. Here we are. Hello, Mrs. Lenning, do you mind if Paula gives you your medication as an assessment?

Mrs. Lenning: No, I don't mind at all.

Paula: Thanks, Mrs. Lenning. OK. I'm going to follow the "five rights" of medication administration for patient safety. Mrs. Lenning is ordered Lasix. Erm, it's in her drawer here as furosemide.

Anna:	Yes, that's the correct drug, but it should have been ordered by its generic name, furosemide, not its brand, or proprietary name, Lasix.
Paula:	Yes, it can be unclear sometimes, can't it? Um, the medication is ordered for Mrs. Eileen Lenning. I'll just check the hospital label on the chart. Mrs. Eileen Lenning, so that's right. If you don't mind, Mrs. Lenning, I'd like to check your identification bracelet, too.
Mrs. Lenning:	Why would you do that? You know who I am.
Paula:	You'd be surprised, Mrs. Lenning. Sometimes two patients with the same name are in the hospital at the same time.
Mrs. Lenning:	Oh, fancy that!
Anna:	What route of administration do you have to use?
Paula:	Oral, I suppose. The doctor hasn't written that in.
Anna:	That's a problem, isn't it? The doctor may want to use the oral route or IV route.
Paula:	Ah, I see what you mean.
Anna:	What about the dose?
Paula:	It's not written in. It's usually 40mg, but the dose would depend on her blood levels.
Anna:	Quite right. You couldn't assume. It could have dangerous consequences.
Paula:	Mm. There's a problem with the frequency and time of administration as well. The doctor hasn't noted down the frequency the medication is to be given or the times. That's a problem, especially with furosemide. It's usually given before midday in divided doses so the patient is not troubled by getting up frequently to go to the toilet in the evening.
Mrs. Lenning:	Thanks for your careful and responsible attitude.
Anna:	That's what we should do. I'll be happy to give this medicine.

🎧 Key Words

assessment / ə'sesmənt / n. 评定，评估
administration / əd,mɪnɪ'streɪʃn / n.（药的）配给；处理
Lasix / 'leɪsɪks / n. 呋喃苯胺酸制剂商品名
drawer / drɔː(r) / n. 抽屉
furosemide / fjʊə'rəʊsəmaɪd / n. 呋喃苯胺酸（强效利尿剂）

generic / dʒə'nerɪk / adj. 非商标的；通用的
proprietary / prə'praɪətri / adj. 专利的
label / 'leɪbl / n. 标签
assume / ə'sjuːm / v. 假定
consequence / 'kɒnsɪkwəns / n. 后果；影响
frequency / 'friːkwənsi / n. 频率；次数

Useful Expressions

identification bracelet　身份手镯
oral route　口服（给药）途径

IV route　静脉（给药）途径

Exercise

I **Read the dialogue again and decide whether the following statements are right or wrong. If there is not enough information to answer "Right" or "Wrong", choose "Doesn't say".**

1. The "five rights" are the right drug, the right patient, the right dose, the right route and the right time. _____.

   A. Right   B. Wrong   C. Doesn't say

2. The drug should have been ordered by its proprietary name, Lasix, NOT its generic name, furosemide. _____.

   A. Right   B. Wrong   C. Doesn't say

3. The doctor has written the medical route of administration. _____.

   A. Right   B. Wrong   C. Doesn't say

4. The dose would depend on Mrs. Lenning's blood pressure and blood glucose. _____.

   A. Right   B. Wrong   C. Doesn't say

5. Anna and Paula are praised for their careful and responsible attitude by Mrs. Lenning. _____.

   A. Right   B. Wrong   C. Doesn't say

II **Discussion.**

What "five rights" should nurses pay attention to when they administer the medications?

Part 2 Short Passage

🎧 Intramuscular Injection

Intramuscular (also IM or im) injection is injecting a medication directly into a muscle, usually the muscle of the upper arm, thigh, or buttock. In medicine, it is one of several alternative methods for the administration of medications. It should be given with extreme care, especially in the buttock, because the sciatic nerve may be injured or a large blood vessel may be entered if the injection is not made correctly into the upper, outer quadrant of the buttock. The deltoid muscle at the shoulder is also used, but less commonly than the gluteus muscle of the buttock; care must be taken to insert the needle in the centre, 2 cm below the acromion. Muscles have larger and more blood vessels than subcutaneous tissue and injections here usually have faster rates of absorption than subcutaneous injections+ or intradermal injections.

[Procedure]

1. Check the medication order.

2. Prepare the correct dosage of the drug from a vial or an ampule.

3. If the medication is particularly irritating to subcutaneous tissue, change the needle on the syringe before the injection.

4. Select the intramuscular site for adequate muscular mass.

5. Establish the exact site for the injection and assist the patient to an appropriate position.

6. Clean the site with an antiseptic swab. Using a circular motion, start at the centre and move outward about 5 cm.

7. Remove the needle cover.

8. Push the syringe and expel any excess air that accidentally entered the syringe.

9. Use the non-dominant hand to spread the skin at the site.

10. Holding the syringe between the thumb and forefinger, pierce the skin quickly at a 90 degree angle, and insert the needle into the muscle.

11. Aspirate by holding the barrel of the syringe steady with the non-dominant hand and by pulling back the plunger with the dominant hand. If blood appears in the syringe, withdraw the needle, discard the syringe, and prepare a new injection. If blood does not appear, inject the medication steadily and slowly, holding the syringe steady.

12. After the injection, apply gentle pressure to the injection site to stop bleeding.

13. Dispose of materials, wash your hands, chart the injection, and observe the patient.

🎧 Key Words

intramuscular /ˌɪntrəˈmʌskjələ(r) / *adj.* 肌内的

sciatic / saɪˈætɪk / *adj.* 坐骨神经的

quadrant / ˈkwɒdrənt / *n.* 四分之一圆

deltoid / ˈdeltɔɪd / *adj.* 三角形的

gluteus / ˈɡluːtiəs / *n.* 臀肌

acromion / əˈkrəʊmjən / *n.* 肩峰

subcutaneous /ˌsʌbkjuˈteɪniəs / *adj.* 皮下的

intradermal /ˌɪntrəˈdɜːməl / *adj.* 皮内的

antiseptic /ˌæntɪˈseptɪk / *adj.* 抗菌的

dominant / ˈdɒmɪnənt / *adj.* 优势的，支配的

aspirate / ˈæspərət / *vt.* 吸入；抽吸

massage / ˈmæsaːʒ / *vt.* 按摩

Useful Expressions

blood vessel　血管

subcutaneous tissue　皮下组织

intradermal injections　皮内注射

thumb and forefinger　拇指和食指

barrel of the syringe　针筒

Exercise

Ⅰ Choose the best answer to each question based on the text.

1. IM injections should be given with extreme care, especially in the buttock, because the _____ may be injured if the injection is not made correctly.

　　A. gluteus muscles　　B. deltoid muscles　　C. sciatic nerve

2. Which of the following positions is NOT commonly used when giving IM injections? _____.

　　A. The deltoid muscle at the shoulder　　B. The muscle of the upper arm and thigh

　　C. The gluteus muscle of the buttock

3. When giving IM injections, pierce the skin quickly at _____, and insert the needle into the muscle.

   A. a 60 degree angle B. a 90 degree angle   C. a 120 degree angle

4. According to the passage, which kind of the following injections has faster rates of absorption?

   A. subcutaneous injection   B. intramuscular injection

   C. intradermal injection

5. The IM injection site is pressed gently _____.

   A. to relieve the pain   B. to irritate the subcutaneous tissue

   C. to stop bleeding

Ⅱ Read the passage again and put the following extracts in the correct order.

   ☐ **A** Select the intramuscular site.

   ☐ **B** Push the syringe and expel any excess air.

   ☐ **C** Insert the needle at a 90 degree angle.

   ☐ **D** Prepare the correct dosage of the drug.

   ☐ **E** Remove the needle cover.

   ☐ **F** Press the injection site gently to stop bleeding.

   ☐ **G** Clean the site with an antiseptic swab.

   ☐ **H** Chart the injection, and observe the patient.

Part 3 Text

🎧 Medication Administration

A medication is a drug administered for its therapeutic effects. Knowledge about the routes of administration is crucial for the health care workers to give medications correctly.

Oral Medications

• Oral Administration

Oral medications are swallowed and must be absorbed into the bloodstream through the intestinal wall by nasogastric feeding tubes or gastrostomy tubes, which is safe, convenient, and acceptable for most clients.

• Sublingual Administration

The sublingual tablet is placed under the tongue, such as nitroglycerin, a medication to treat angina pectoris.

Parenteral Medications

The parenteral route means that medications are given by injection or infusion. Parenteral medications may be injected into intradermal (ID), subcutaneous (SC), or intramuscular tissue; into intravenous or intra-arterial circulation.

• Intradermal Injections

Intradermal injections are given into the dermis, which the layer of tissue is located beneath the skin surface, and are commonly used for allergy testing. They are usually administered into the inner forearm area.

- **Subcutaneous Injections**

Subcutaneous injections are given into the SC tissue, the layer of fat located below the dermis and above the muscle tissue. They may be given in the upper arm, upper back, abdomen, upper buttocks, or thigh.

- **Intramuscular Injections**

Intramuscular injections are given into the muscle layer beneath the dermis and SC tissue. Medications administered by IM injection are usually absorbed intermediately, slower than IV administration but more rapidly than SC injection. IM injections may be administered into sites in the upper arm, hip or thigh.

- **Intravenous Administration**

Intravenous medications are given by way of catheters inserted into veins. IV catheters can be placed in the peripheral or the central circulation. Good technical skill is needed in administering this injection. IV medications must be prepared and packaged in a sterile manner to prevent infection. Leakage of medications into surrounding tissues may result in damage to tissues.

Topical Medications

Topical medications are placed on the skin surface or mucous membranes. They may also be placed in body cavities. Ophthalmic solutions and ointments may be used to treat eye irritation, infections. Otic solutions can be dropped into the ear to treat external ear infections. Nasal solutions are usually sprayed into the nose to treat nasal congestion. Rectal medications in suppository form may be placed in the rectum to treat systemic complaints or as a laxative to encourage bowel movements. Vaginal medications may be used for contraception, to help kill bacteria before gynecologic surgery, or to treat vaginal infection.

Inhaled Medications

Inhaled medications may be used to treat respiratory disorders or to induce anaesthesia during surgery. Inhalation is often administered by nebulizers. The frequently used types of nebulization are handheld nebulization, oxygen nebulization and ultrasonic nebulization.

There are some common abbreviations used in the medication orders.

Abbreviation Form

Medication Administration		Dosage Forms		Administration Time	
IM	intramuscular	cap., caps.	capsule	a.c.	before meals
IV	intravenous	inj.	injection	bid	twice a day
PO	by mouth	tab.	tablet	p.c.	after meals
				prn	as needed according to necessity
				qd	every day
				q4h	every four hours
				qid	four times a day
				tid	three times a day

🎧 Key Words

nasogastric /ˌneɪzəʊ'ɡæstrɪk/ *adj.* 鼻饲的

gastrostomy /ɡæs'trɒstəmi/ *n.* 胃造口术

sublingual /sʌb'lɪŋɡwəl/ *adj.* 舌下的

nitroglycerin /ˌnaɪtrəʊ'ɡlɪsərɪn/ *n.* 硝酸甘油

parenteral /pə'rentərəl/ *adj.* 肠胃外的；不经肠道的

intra-arterial /'ɪntrə ɑː'tɪəriəl/ *adj.* 动脉内的

peripheral /pə'rɪfərəl/ *adj.*（神经）末梢区域的

ophthalmic /ɒf'θælmɪk/ *adj.* 眼睛的

ointment /'ɔɪntmənt/ *n.* 药膏

suppository /sə'pɒzətri/ *n.* 栓剂

laxative /'læksətɪv/ *n.* 泻药

vaginal /və'dʒaɪnl/ *adj.* 阴道的

contraception /ˌkɒntrə'sepʃn/ *n.* 避孕

nebulizer /'nebjʊlaɪzə/ *n.* 喷雾器

ultrasonic /ˌʌltrə'sɒnɪk/ *adj.* 超声的

Useful Expressions

angina pectoris　心绞痛

mucous membrane　黏膜

body cavity　体腔

gynecologic surgery　妇科手术

respiratory disorders　呼吸道疾病

Exercise

I　Choose the best answer to each question based on the text.

1. How many types of topical medications are introduced in the section of Topical Medications?
   _____.
   A. Three　　　　　　　　B. Four　　　　　　　　C. Five

2. Oral medications can be administrated by _____.
   A. oral route and subcutaneous injection
   B. oral route and intramuscular injection
   C. oral route and sublingual route

3. How can parenteral medications be administered? _____.
   A. By oral route
   B. By injection or infusion
   C. By nebulizers

4. Generally speaking, medications administered by _____ are absorbed fastest.
   A. IV injection　　　　　B. SC injection　　　　　C. IM injection

5. _____ can be dropped into the ear to treat external ear infections.
   A. Otic solutions　　　　B. Ophthalmic ointments　　　　C. Nasal solutions

II　Match each medical term in Column A with its explanation in Column B.

Column A	Column B
_____　1. gastrostomy	a. under the tongue
_____　2. sublingual	b. below the epidermis

_____	3. subcutaneous	c. a surgical opening into the stomach
_____	4. ophthalmic	d. methods of preventing pregnancy
_____	5. contraception	e. relating to or concerned with people's eyes

Ⅲ Find words or terms in the article to match the following definitions.

1. a food or drug that stimulates evacuation of the bowels _____
2. a dispenser that turns a liquid into a fine mist _____
3. of or relating to the nose and stomach _____
4. entering the body not by the alimentary tract but by another means _____

Ⅳ Critical thinking.

According to the case at the beginning of this unit, what are the "five rights" of medication administration for patient safety?

Nurses should follow the "five rights" of medication administration when doing the assessment. The right drug: crosscheck the name of medication on the Presciption Chart and the medication label. The drug should be ordered by its generic name. The right patient: check the patient's full name by checking the hospital label and the patient's identification bracelet. The right dose: crosscheck the dose of medication, and adjustment needs to be made according to patient's blood level. The right route: check the route of medication on the Chart. The common routes are: IV, IM, and oral route. The right time: check the frequency and time of administration.

Part 4 Supplementary Reading

🎧 Skin Allergy Test

Skin allergy test is a method for medical diagnosis of allergies that attempts to provoke a small, controlled, allergic response. Information from allergy tests may help the doctor develop an allergy treatment plan that includes allergen avoidance, medications or allergy shots (immunotherapy).

Skin allergy tests are widely used to help diagnose allergic conditions, including:

- Hay fever (allergic rhinitis)
- Allergic asthma
- Dermatitis (eczema)
- Food allergies
- Penicillin allergy
- Bee venom allergy
- Latex allergy

Skin tests are generally safe for adults and children of all ages, including infants. In certain circumstances, though, skin tests aren't recommended. The doctors may advise against skin testing if patients:

- Have ever had a severe allergic reaction. Patients may be so sensitive to certain substances that even the tiny amounts used in skin tests could trigger a life-threatening reaction (anaphylaxis).

- Take medications that could interfere with test results. These include antihistamines, many antidepressants and some heartburn medications. The doctor may determine that it's better for patients to continue taking these medications than to temporarily discontinue them in preparation for a skin test.

- Have certain skin conditions. If severe eczema or psoriasis affects large areas of skin on the patient's arms and back—the usual testing sites—there may not be enough clear, uninvolved skin to do an effective test. Other skin conditions, such as dermographism, can cause unreliable test results.

The most common side effect of skin testing is slightly swollen, red, itchy bumps (wheals). Some allergies are identified in a few minutes but others may take several days. In all cases where the test is positive, the skin will become raised, red and appear itchy. The results are recorded—larger wheals indicating that the subject is more sensitive to that particular allergen. A negative test does not conclusively rule out an allergy; occasionally, the concentration needs to be adjusted, or the body fails to elicit a response.

Clients who undergo skin testing should know that anaphylaxis can occur anytime. So if any of the following symptoms are experienced, a physician consultation is recommended immediately:

- Low grade fever
- Lightheadedness or dizziness
- Wheezing or shortness of breath
- Extensive skin rash
- Swelling of face, lips or mouth
- Difficulty swallowing or speaking

Exercise

Choose the best answer to each question based on the text.

1. According to the passage, skin allergy tests are widely used to help diagnose allergic conditions, including _____.

   A. allergic rhinitis and allergic asthma

   B. penicillin allergy and allergic bronchitis

   C. allergic dermatitis and dermal ulcer

2. According to the passage, the doctor may NOT recommend the skin allergy test if patients _____.

   A. have ever had severe allergic reaction

   B. have ever had severe asthma

   C. have ever had severe dermatitis

3. According to the passage, the following medications could interfere with skin allergy test results except _____.

   A. antihistamine   B. antidepressant   C. antimicrobial

4. In all cases where the test is _____, the skin will become raised, red and appear itchy.

    A. positive   B. negative   C. neutral

5. _____ are identified in a few minutes after the skin allergy test is given.

    A. All allergies   B. Some allergies   C. Many allergies

Part 5 Medical Word Elements

1. amin(o)-   氨基
   aminoacidemia / ˌæmɪnəʊˌæsɪˈdiːmɪə /   氨基酸血症
   aminophylline / ˌæmɪnəʊˈfɪliːn /   氨茶碱

2. chlor(o)-   氯
   chloride / ˈklɔːraɪd /   氯化物
   chlorpromazine / klɔːˈprəʊməziːn /   氯丙嗪

3. de-   除去
   deacetylation / dɪəsɪtɪˈleɪʃən /   脱乙酰作用
   deoxyribose / diːˌɒksɪˈraɪbəʊs /   脱氧核糖

4. dextr(o)-   右旋的
   dextrose / ˈdekstrəʊs /   葡萄糖，右旋糖
   dextran / ˈdekstrən /   右旋糖酐，葡聚糖

5. hydr(o)-   水，氢
   hydroxide / haɪˈdrɒksaɪd /   羟化物，氢氧化物
   hydrochloride / ˌhaɪdrəˈkləʊraɪd /   盐酸化物，盐酸盐

6. albumin(o)-   白蛋白
   albuminolysis / ælˌbjʊmɪˈnɒlɪsɪs /   白蛋白分解
   albuminuria / ˌælbjʊmɪnˈjʊərɪə /   白蛋白尿，蛋白尿

7. nitro-, nitra   硝基
   nitrazepam / naɪˈtræzɪpæm /   硝基安定
   nitrogen / ˈnaɪtrədʒən /   氮

8. calc(i)-   钙的，钙盐的
   calcitonin / ˌkælsɪˈtəʊnɪn /   降钙素
   calcium / ˈkælsɪəm /   钙

9. oxy-   化合物内有氧存在
   oxygenase / ˈɒksɪdʒɪˌneɪs /   加氧酶
   oxyhemoglobin / ˌɒksɪˈhiːməˌgləʊbɪn /   氧合血红蛋白

（王炎峰　赵　静）

Wound Care

Learning Objectives:

1. *Discussing wound assessment with patients*
2. *Describing the practice of aseptic technique*
3. *Explaining the wound management*
4. *Investigating the different types of dressings*

Lead-In

Case Study

Mr. Smith was a 56-year-old smoker with a long history of Peripheral Vascular Disease. Three months ago, he developed a venous ulcer on his left ankle after he slipped on the stairs. His local doctor asked the district nurse to come and dress the wound at home. Two days ago he was admitted to hospital to assess his circulation and monitor wound management. The result showed that he had a poor blood circulation in his lower legs. Signs and symptoms showed that the wound was quite sore and the surrounding skin had become red. His body temperature was 38.1 ℃ .

Part 1 Dialogue

🎧 Wound Assessment

David Parker, the clinical nurse specialist, is making his usual rounds in the morning. The patient's son claimed that the gauze on the patient's wound had been soaked and wanted to change the dressing. Emily, the nurse, is examining the patient.

David: Hello, Mr. Smith. I am David Parker. I'm the clinical nurse specialist here.

Mr. Smith: Oh. Hello, Mr. Parker.

David: I believe you must have a rough time with long-term half sitting in wheelchair. Since you can't move easily, Emily will examine your buttocks quickly.

Emily: Now, I'll take off your dressing. Tell me if I hurt you too much.

Mr. Smith: Oh, OK, take your time.

David: Would you mind if you tell me something about the nursing management at home?

Mr. Smith: Oh, as you know, after cerebrovascular accident, life has been hard on me; I need quite a lot of help. However my wife died last year, my children have to take leaves to take care of me day and night. I think I am a heavy burden on them.

David: But have you thought that they did this because of their love and hope for you? They hope you'll recover better someday.

Mr. Smith: Perhaps you're right, but I am always feeling anxious.

David: Take it easy. Tell me what do you usually eat at home?

Mr. Smith: I don't have a good appetite. Most of the time, I eat vegetables and noodles.

David: Your diet is too light. You need high-calorie, high-protein things to increase your nutrition, such as eggs, milk, lean meat, fish, and shrimp. Vitamin C and zinc are also good for your health. Do you agree with me?

Mr. Smith: I'll try my best.

David: Emily, how is the wound?

Emily: It's a chronic infection wound. The wound is on the sacrococcygeal region. There is a lot of ooze and it smells a bit. Black necrosis can be seen in the centre circle, the base of the wound is 75% yellow and 25% red. The wound size is 7.5 cm × 6.1 cm × 2.3 cm. The surrounding skin is red and swollen. The edge of the wound is irregular.

David: Er, I see. It is a stage-IV pressure ulcer. Well, I'd like to use a VAC dressing on this wound.

Mr. Smith: Oh. Sounds disgusting.

David: Mr. Smith, the VAC means vacuum-assisted closure, but it's only a gentle suction on the wound.

Mr. Smith: I see. Do you think it'll be a good method to help the wound heal faster?

David: Yes. The continued vacuum draws out fluid from the wound and increases blood flow to the area to promote wound healing.

Mr. Smith: Sounds like a good idea. By the way, my clothes are all wet from sweating during the night. Can I have it changed now?

David: Of course. Emily will bring the clean one for you. She'll help you to change.

Mr. Smith: Fine.

David: Emily, be sure to turn over the patient every two hours. Every day use warm water to scrub the whole body and change clothes in time.

Emily: Yes, Mr. Parker.

🎧 Key Words

dressing / ˈdresɪŋ / n. 敷料；绷带
buttock / ˈbʌtək / n. 臀部
cerebrovascular / ˌserəbrəʊˈvæskjələ(r) / adj. 脑血管的

protein / ˈprəʊtiːn / n. 蛋白质
zinc / zɪŋk / n. 锌
sacrococcygeal / ˌsækrəˈkɒksɪdʒiːl / adj. 骶尾的

necrosis / ne'krəʊsɪs / n.（细胞组织）坏死　　　suction / 'sʌkʃn / n. 抽吸

ulcer / 'ʌlsə(r) / n. 溃疡；腐烂物

Useful Expressions

wound assessment　伤口评估　　　　　　pressure ulcer　压疮

chronic wound　慢性伤口　　　　　　　vacuum-assisted closure (VAC)　封闭式负压引流

Exercise

I **Read the dialogue again and decide whether the following statements are right or wrong. If there is not enough information to answer "Right" or "Wrong", choose "Doesn't say".**

1. The nurse is talking with Mr. Smith about wound assessment. _____.
   A. Right　　　　　　B. Wrong　　　　　　C. Doesn't say
2. Mr. Smith has a good control of his body. _____.
   A. Right　　　　　　B. Wrong　　　　　　C. Doesn't say
3. Mr. Smith has a light diet. _____.
   A. Right　　　　　　B. Wrong　　　　　　C. Doesn't say
4. VAC dressing can promote the wound healing. _____.
   A. Right　　　　　　B. Wrong　　　　　　C. Doesn't say
5. Mr. Smith will be discharged soon. _____.
   A. Right　　　　　　B. Wrong　　　　　　C. Doesn't say

II **Discussion.**

How does Mr. Smith cooperate with the nurse while in the hospital?

Part 2 Short Passage

🎧 Aseptic Technique

Aseptic technique refers to a series of operation techniques in the process of medical care operation to keep sterile articles and sterile areas free from contamination and to prevent pathogenic microorganisms from invading the human body. This can be achieved by ensuring that only sterile equipment and fluids are used during invasive medical and nursing procedures.

Aseptic technique includes a series of steps that complement each other.

1. Personal preparation. Wash hands and wear clean clothes, hats, and masks. When wearing a mask, keep it close to your face and cover your nose, mouth and chin completely.

2. Spread the sterile towel. Open the sterile bag and use an aseptic clipper to place a treatment towel in the treatment tray; if the package is not used up, wrap the original creases and mark the date and time of the package. Hold the two corners of the sterile towel with both hands and gently shake off. Half of the treatment towel is placed on the treatment plate, and the upper and lower sides are aligned to the upper part of the upper quadrant three times, and the outside of the opening is outward, making the inner surface of the treatment towel a sterile area.

3. Pick up items. Open the sterile bag, sterile cotton ball and gauze can, and put the required sterile articles into the sterile towel; take a sterile solution.

4. Fold aseptic bag. Align the lower layer of the treatment towel, fold the opening up twice, and fold down the edges of both sides to reveal the edge of the treatment plate.

5. Label. If the aseptic dish is not used immediately, mark the name and time of the item on the card, place it on the prepared treatment plate, and arrange the other items.

6. Wear sterile gloves. Check the gloves before you open them, take out the glove by holding the folding part (inside), and put the glove on the other hand. The gloved fingers are inserted into the fold of the other glove (outside), and the glove is worn. Place the folding part of the gloves over the sleeves. Rinse the talcum powder on the gloves with sterile saline. When wearing gloves, the outside of gloves should not touch the inner surface of gloves and non-sterile items or areas. If gloves are damaged or contaminated, they should be replaced immediately. Wash the blood stains before removing the gloves. When one gloved hand is turned over and removed, it will insert into the inside of the other glove. It is flipped out and placed in the medical waste bin, which is pushed to the disposal room to be classified and processed.

🎧 Key Words

aseptic / ˌeɪ'septɪk / adj. 无菌的；防腐性的
pathogenic / ˌpæθə'dʒenɪk / adj. 致病的；病原的
tray / treɪ / n. 托盘
crease / kri:s / n. 折痕；折缝

contamination / kənˌtæmɪ'neɪʃn / n. 污染；污染物
align / ə'laɪn / v. 排列；排成一行
gauze / gɔ:z / n. 纱布

Useful Expressions

aseptic technique　无菌操作法
aseptic clipper　无菌持物钳

sterile towel　治疗巾
disposal room　处置室

Exercise

I Choose the best answer to each question based on the text.

1. The correct way to wear a mask is covering your _____ completely.

　　A. mouth and nose　　B. mouth and chin　　C. mouth, nose and chin

2. Which of the following is wrong when performing aseptic technique? _____.

　　A. Use an aseptic clipper to place a treatment towel

　　B. Fold the opening part of the treatment towel and both sides

C. Use hands to take sterile items directly

3. When an item in a sterile bag is NOT used up, the nurse should NOT _____.

    A. wrap the original creases

    B. mark the date and time of the package

    C. throw them away after 6 hours

4. If gloves are found to be damaged or contaminated, the doctors and nurses should _____.

    A. disinfect them immediately

    B. replace them immediately

    C. stop the operation immediately

5. When the doctors and nurses are removing the gloves, the best way is to _____.

    A. take them off no matter whether the gloves are polluted or not

    B. pull the finger down first

    C. turn over the gloves on the wrist and remove them

II Read the passage again and put the following extracts in the correct order.

    ☐ **A** Take out the glove by holding the folding part (inside).

    ☐ **B** The gloved fingers are inserted into the fold of the other glove (outside).

    ☐ **C** Check the gloves.

    ☐ **D** Put the glove on the other hand.

    ☐ **E** Place the folding part of the gloves over the sleeves.

    ☐ **F** Rinse the talcum powder on the gloves with sterile saline.

Part 3 Text

🎧 Wound

In pathology, wound specifically refers to a sharp injury which damages the dermis of the skin. The degree of contamination in the wound itself is strongly associated with subsequent infection, and a widely accepted method of classification is as follows: clean-wound, clean-contaminated wound, contaminated wound and dirty or infected wound.

According to the colour of the wound, the red wound indicates normal healing; the yellow wound indicates that there is slough, exudate or infection in the wound; black is the most unhealthy skin colour, marking necrosis. There are two or even three colours in a mixed wound, find the unhealthiest colour, and then classify the wound as the unhealthiest colour cut.

Wound is also classified by the length of healing time: acute and chronic wound. Acute wound mainly means minor wounds, will heal on their own in one or two weeks. Chronic wound is a wound that does not heal in an orderly set of stages the way most wounds do. The vast majority of chronic wounds can be classified into three categories: venous ulcer, diabetic, and pressure ulcer.

Some scientists have found that chronic wounds contain unusually high levels of protease and pro-inflammatory cytokines, and prolonged inflammation is considered the most significant factor in delayed healing. Wound bed preparation (WBP) is a systematic approach to correct molecular and cellular abnormalities; it includes four key principles, the TIME principle: tissue debridement, inflammation, moisture balance and edge of the wound.

There are several types of debridement: surgical debridement, conservation sharp wound debridement, larval debridement, chemical debridement, autolytic debridement and mechanical debridement (wet to dry dressing, irrigation under pressure). In clinical practice, one or two methods of debridement are often selected in accordance with the patient's wound. When the patient is in a poor body condition, conservative surgical debridement or mechanical debridement can be adopted first; then hydrogel dressing can be used for autolyzed debridement. It can achieve the purpose of quickly debridement, and guarantee the effect of radical debridement. It's important to note that the wound should be assessed before debridement; when the wound is at the end of the limb, the peripheral blood flow should be evaluated first; re-evaluate the wound each time when the dressing is changed.

The treatment of infected wounds should adhere to strict aseptic operation. To lower the bacterial load in wounds, therapists may use topical antibiotics. They can kill bacteria and keep the wound environment moist, which is important for speeding the healing of chronic wounds. Excessive fluid in chronic wound can interfere with the activities of important cell mediators such as growth factors in the tissue. The management goal is to promote moisture balance in wounds and to choose an appropriate dressing.

Negative pressure wound therapy (NPWT) is a treatment that improves ischemic tissues and removes wound fluid used by bacteria. This therapy, also known as vacuum-assisted closure, reduces swelling in tissues, which brings more blood and nutrients to the area. This treatment is applicable to the following symptoms: chronic open wounds, flaps and grafts, dehisced wounds, diabetic ulcers, pressure ulcers, acute and traumatic wounds, partial thickness burns, etc.

Absorbent dressings can also be used to properly control the moist environment. When there is a small amount of infiltration, <5 ml/d, or gauze dressing is changed once a day, film and hydrogel can be chosen for the wound. When the amount of infiltration is up to 5-10 ml/d, or gauze dressing is changed twice or three times a day, hydrocolloid and alginate can be used. When there is a lot of infiltration, >10 ml/d, or gauze dressing is changed more than three times a day, foam is the best option.

Although the treatment and nursing of chronic wound is very important, it is more important to pay attention to the home rehabilitation and prevention of recurrence after discharge.

🎧 Key Words

dermis / 'dɜːmɪs / n. 皮肤，真皮	debridement / dɪ'brɪdmənt / n. 清创术
protease / 'prəʊtɪeɪz / n. 蛋白酶	larval / 'lɑːvl / adj. 幼虫的
cytokine / ˌsɪtə'kɪn / n. 细胞活素	graft / grɑːft / n. 移植
slough / slʌf / n. 腐肉	dehisce / dɪ'hɪs / vi.（伤口）裂开
exudate / 'eksjudeɪt / n. 分泌液；渗出物	traumatic / trɔː'mætɪk / adj. 创伤的
inflammation / ˌɪnflə'meɪʃn / n. 炎症	rehabilitation / ˌriːəˌbɪlɪ'teɪʃn / n. 康复

Useful Expressions

clean-contaminated wound　半污染伤口	wound fluid　创面积液，伤口渗出液
acute wound　急性伤口	negative pressure wound therapy (NPWT)
bacterial load　细菌负荷	伤口负压治疗法
topical antibiotics　外用抗生素	

Exercise

▮ Choose the best answer to each question based on the text.

1. How many types of chronic wound does the text mention? _____.

　　A. 2　　　　　　　　B. 3　　　　　　　　C. 4

2. If a wound has two colours: red and yellow, it is a _____ wound.

　　A. yellow　　　　　　B. red　　　　　　　C. black

3. In order to speed the wound healing, the nurse should keep the wound environment _____.

　　A. moist　　　　　　B. dry　　　　　　　C. anaerobic

4. The role of NPWT is to _____.

　　A. improve ischemic tissues

　　B. remove wound fluid

　　C. both A and B

5. What is the most important factor that affects wound healing? _____.

　　A. Contamination　　B. Bacteria　　　　　C. Inflammation

▮▮ Match each medical term in Column A with its explanation in Column B.

	Column A	Column B
_____	1. swelling	a. necrotic tissue
_____	2. ischemia	b. abnormal protuberance
_____	3. dehisce	c. local anaemia
_____	4. exudate	d. a substance that oozes out from pores
_____	5. slough	e. burst or split open

III Find words or terms in the article to match the following definitions.

1. surgical removal of foreign material and dead tissue from a wound _____

2. a wound when it is made dirty or infected by germs _____

3. a response of body tissues to injury or irritation; characterized by pain and swelling and redness and heat _____

4. of or relating to self-digestion, refers to the destruction of a cell through the action of its own enzymes _____

IV Critical thinking.

According to the case at the beginning of this unit, what are nursing diagnoses and nursing interventions for the patient?

1. Nursing diagnoses

- Risk for infection related to the wound
- Impaired skin integrity related to the injury
- Hyperthermia related to the infections

2. Nursing interventions

The patient should be started on some antibiotic therapy to stop the infection. The VAC (Vacuum-Assisted Closure) dressing will help the wound heal faster. Education about maintaining regular lifestyle is critical. To prevent further deterioration of the ulcer, the patient should quit smoking due to poor blood circulation.

Part 4 Supplementary Reading

🎧 Dressings

A dressing is a sterile pad or compress applied to a wound to promote healing and protect the wound from further harm. A dressing is designed to be in direct contact with the wound, as distinguished from a bandage, which is most often used to hold a dressing in place. Many modern dressings are self-adhesive, they are produced as an "island" surrounded by an adhesive backing, ready for immediate application—these are known as island dressings.

Modern dressings mainly include gauze dressing, alginate dressing, transparent film dressing, hydrocolloid dressing, antibiotic and bioelectric dressing.

The traditional gauze dressing is the most commonly used dressing due to their simplicity and inexpensiveness. It is made from an open-weave fabric, cotton. It cannot be used for infective wound which has no promoting effect to wound healing. Today, gauze dressing often has a layer of non-stick, perforated plastic film over the absorbent gauze to prevent excessive drying of a wound or adhesion to the dressing, but maintaining the gauze's ability to absorb exudate. Non-stick gauze island dressing is the most common type of dressing today—an example is the Band-Aid.

Alginate dressing is one of the most advanced medical dressings. The main ingredient of alginate dressing is alginate, which is a natural polysaccharide carbohydrate extracted from seaweed, which is a kind of natural cellulose. It can absorb up to twenty times the weight of its liquid. After the medical film is exposed to the wound exudation, it can form a soft gel to provide an ideal moist environment to promote wound healing and alleviate the pain of the wound. However most products are not self-adhesive and need to be fixed with supplementary dressing.

Transparent film dressing does not absorb exudate, they are regarded to exchange oxygen and water vapour and maintain the optimum temperature to encourage healing. However liquids and bacteria can't penetrate. The wound can be directly observed through transparent film dressing which mechanically debrides a wound by removing the slough.

Hydrocolloid dressing is made of carbohydrate, which is sticky and plastic, and can't penetrate oxygen, water or water vapour. It can maintain the moist environment of the wound and promote the self-soluble debridement.

Antibiotic is also often used with dressings to prevent bacterial infection. Bioelectric dressing can be effective in attacking certain antibiotic-resistant bacteria and speeding up the healing process.

Exercise

Choose the best answer to each question based on the text.

1. What is the advantage of gauze dressing? _____.

   A. It can absorb exudate

   B. It can promote excessive drying of a wound

   C. It can promote adhesion

2. If there is a large amount of fluid in the wound, which of the following dressings is suitable? _____.

   A. Alginate dressing

   B. Transparent film dressing

   C. Hydrocolloid dressing

3. What is the advantage of transparent film dressing? _____.

   A. It can penetrate liquids

   B. It can exchange oxygen and water vapour

   C. It can absorb exudate

4. Hydrocolloid dressing has the characteristics that _____.

   A. it can't penetrate oxygen, water or water vapour

   B. it can promote self-soluble debridement

   C. Both A and B

5. Which of the following statements is NOT true about bioelectric dressing? _____.

   A. It can attack certain antibiotic-resistant bacteria

   B. It can cause bacterial infection

   C. It can promote healing process

Part 5 Medical Word Elements

1. acr(o)-	肢端，尖端
acromegaly / ˌækrəˈmegəlɪ /	肢端肥大症
acrosclerosis / ˌækrəʊskləˈrəʊsɪs /	肢端硬皮病
2. -penia	减少
thrombopenia / ˌθrɒmbəʊˈpiːnɪə /	血小板减少（症）
leukopenia / ˌluːkəˈpiːnɪə /	白细胞减少（症）
3. fibr(o)-	纤维
fibrinogen / faɪˈbrɪnədʒən /	纤维蛋白原
fibroblast / ˈfaɪbrəblæst /	成纤维细胞
4. py(o)-	脓
pyoderma / ˌpaɪəʊˈdɜːmə /	脓皮病
pyonephritis / ˌpaɪəʊnɪˈfraɪtɪs /	脓性肾炎
5. myc(o)-	真菌
mycobacteria / ˌmiːkəʊbækˈtɪərɪə /	分枝杆菌
mycosis / maɪˈkəʊsɪs /	真菌病
6. cry(o)-	冷，寒冷
crymotherapy / ˌkraɪməʊˈθerəpi /	冷疗法
cryopathy / kraɪˈɒpəθi /	寒冷病
7. erythr(o)-	红，红细胞
erythromycin / ɪˌrɪθrəˈmaɪsɪn /	红霉素
erythrocyte / ɪˈrɪθrəsaɪt /	红细胞
8. leuk(o)-	白，白细胞
leukemia / luːˈkiːmiə /	白血病
leukocyte / ˈluːkəsaɪt /	白细胞
9. cycl(o)-	环，睫状体
cyclectomy / saɪˈlektəmi /	睫状体切开术
cyclosporine / ˌsaɪkləʊˈspɒriːn /	环孢素

（李　静　赵　静）

Medical Specimen

Learning Objectives:

1. *Discussing urine sample collection with patients*
2. *Describing the process of obtaining venous blood*
3. *Defining and classifying the different types of laboratory tests*
4. *Explaining the importance of accurate sample collection*

Lead-In

Case Study

Mrs. Truman was a 48-year-old housewife who came to the clinic to have some tests done. She complained of frequency, urgency and pain when passing urine. Physical examination showed that her face was badly swollen and there was obvious pain around the kidney area. Other symptoms included loss of appetite, fatigue and pale. The nurse suspected that she had got a urinary tract infection, so she was asked to do a urine specimen test to see if there was any bacteria in the urine.

Part 1 Dialogue

🎧 Collecting Midstream Specimen of Urine (MSU)

Rita, a ward nurse, is teaching Mrs. Truman, a patient, to collect midstream urine.

Rita:　　　　Good morning, Mrs. Truman. I'm Rita, the ward nurse. How are you today?

Mrs. Truman: Good morning. Everything goes well, but I feel a bit cold.

Rita:　　　　Oh, I'll get you a blanket later on.

Mrs. Truman: Thank you. You're always very helpful.

Rita:　　　　You're welcome. The morning nurse mentioned in the handover that you passed blood in your urine last night.

Mrs. Truman: Yes, that's awful.

Rita:　　　　The doctor would like you to do a urine specimen test this morning to see if there is any infection in your urinary tract.

Mrs. Truman: OK.

Rita: I've got everything here to do the MSU.

Mrs. Truman: What is MSU?

Rita: It's a short term for midstream specimen of urine. That's to say, your specimen of urine sample comes from the middle part of your urine.

Mrs. Truman: Why is the middle part?

Rita: Because there is less contamination in it. The beginning and the end may influence the result.

Mrs. Truman: Oh. What do I do?

Rita: You need to wash your hands before you go to the toilet. Here is a plastic jar and a specimen container. When you pass urine into the toilet, try to catch the middle part of the stream with the jar and pour the urine stream into the specimen container. When you do this, please do not touch the inside of the jar and the specimen container.

Mrs. Truman: Oh. It's a bit complicated. Shall I give the jar and the specimen container back to you?

Rita: When it's finished, you can throw away the jar into the bin and leave the specimen container on the shelf outside the toilet. Porters will collect it and send it to the lab.

Mrs. Truman: OK.

Rita: Here you are, the jar and the specimen container. Can you repeat the process back to me?

Mrs. Truman: Wash my hands thoroughly. Catch the midstream and pour into the container.

Rita: Right, the midstream of the urine.

Mrs. Truman: OK. The middle part of the urine stream.

Rita: Buzz me if you have any question. See you later.

Mrs. Truman: Yes, I will. Thanks.

🎧 Key Words

specimen / ˈspesɪmən / n.（尿、细胞组织等的）试样，抽样

urine / ˈjʊərɪn / n. 尿

midstream / ˌmɪdˈstriːm / adj.（小便）排至一半时的

urinary / ˈjʊərɪnəri / adj. 尿的；泌尿的

tract / trækt / n. 道；系统

infection / ɪnˈfekʃn / n. 感染；传染

container / kənˈteɪnə(r) / n. 容器

porter / ˈpɔːtə(r) / n. 护工

Useful Expressions

midstream specimen of urine (MSU)   中段尿液样本

urine specimen test   尿样检测

urinary tract   尿道

plastic jar   塑料尿杯

specimen container   样本容器

Exercise

I **Read the dialogue again and decide whether the following statements are right or wrong. If there is not enough information to answer "Right" or "Wrong", choose "Doesn't say".**

1. The nurse is talking with Mrs. Truman about how to collect midstream urine. _____.

   A. Right   B. Wrong   C. Doesn't say

2. Nothing went wrong when Mrs. Truman urinated last night. _____.

   A. Right   B. Wrong   C. Doesn't say

3. Mrs. Truman has infection in her urinary tract. _____.

   A. Right   B. Wrong   C. Doesn't say

4. Mrs. Truman knows MSU and how to collect it. _____.

   A. Right   B. Wrong   C. Doesn't say

5. Mrs. Truman herself should take her urine sample to the lab. _____.

   A. Right   B. Wrong   C. Doesn't say

II **Discussion.**

What are the proper steps to collect MSU?

Part 2 Short Passage

🎧 Venipuncture for Blood

Blood analysis is now carried on in most hospitals around the world to diagnose diseases. One important way to obtain blood from the human body is through venipuncture. Venipuncture is a process during which a health care worker draw blood from a patient's vein located on the inside of the elbow or the back of the hand with certain equipment.

The equipment used for blood collection varied with the age of the patient. Evacuated tube system (ETS) which mainly consists of a needle and evacuated tubes is the most common method used in the U.S. and U.K. Blood test with ETS is performed with the following steps.

1. The site is sterilized with Betadine.

2. An elastic band is tied around the upper arm of the patient to apply pressure to the area.

3. A syringe with a butterfly needle on one end is inserted into the patient's vein.

4. The needle on the other end of the syringe is inserted into the evacuated tube and the vacuum in the tube automatically draws blood into the tube.

5. Multiple evacuated tubes can be applied in turn to draw blood for various diagnostic purposes.

6. When collection is done, the elastic band can be removed.

7. Take out the needle and cover the spot with a bandage. The patient is required to press lightly on the bandage to help the blood clot and to prevent bruising.

Although there is more than one way of blood drawing, venipuncture is preferred in the pathology department. There are a number of advantages.

1. Venipuncture allows a much more volume of blood collection without any danger to the patient.

2. Venipuncture is a good way of blood storage for future additional tests.

3. Venipuncture is much more flexible when it comes to puncture site selection.

4. The patient feels less painful with venipuncture.

5. Venipuncture is the only way of collection for some special tests.

6. The results of venipuncture are more reliable.

With the above advantages, venipuncture is no doubt an ideal method of blood collection for adults. However, when applied to infants, some other methods may be preferable.

🎧 Key Words

venipuncture / ˈvenɪˌpʌŋktʃə / n. 静脉穿刺
vein / veɪn / n. 静脉
evacuate / ɪˈvækjueɪt / vt. 抽空
sterilize / ˈsterəlaɪz / vt. 消毒
Betadine / ˈbetədɪn / n. 必妥碘（药物品牌名）
elastic / ɪˈlæstɪk / adj. 有弹性的

vacuum / ˈvækjuːm / n. 真空
automatically / ˌɔːtəˈmætɪkli / adv. 自动地
bandage / ˈbændɪdʒ / n. 绷带
bruising / ˈbruːzɪŋ / n. 挫伤
pathology / pəˈθɒlədʒi / n. 病理学

Useful Expressions

blood analysis   血液分析
evacuated tube system (ETS)   真空管系统

blood test   血液检测

Exercise

Ⅰ Choose the best answer to each question based on the text.

1. One important way to obtain blood from the human body is through _____.

    A. acupuncture   B. venipuncture   C. injection

2. Which of the following is NOT included in an evacuated tube system (ETS)? _____.

    A. A needle   B. Evacuated tubes   C. Betadine

3. What helps drawing the blood automatically into the tubes? _____.

    A. The needle   B. The vacuum   C. The nurse

4. What is the patient required to do after the needle is taken out? _____.

    A. Press lightly on the bandage

    B. Take off the bandage

    C. Wash hands

5. What is the advantage of venipuncture? _____.

    A. The patient feels more painful

    B. The results change from time to time

    C. It is a good way for blood storage

II **Read the passage again and put the following extracts in the correct order.**

☐ **A** Multiple evacuated tubes can be applied in turn to draw blood.

☐ **B** An elastic band is tied around the upper arm of the patient.

☐ **C** Take out the needle and cover the spot with a bandage.

☐ **D** A syringe with a butterfly needle on one end is inserted into the patient's vein.

☐ **E** The site is sterilized with Betadine.

☐ **F** Remove the elastic band.

☐ **G** The needle on the other end of the syringe is inserted into the evacuated tube.

Part 3 Text

🎧 Medical Specimens

Medical laboratory is a department which is commonly seen in most hospitals and also known as the pathology department. Hundreds of tests are done every day on the specimens provided by the patients to obtain information about their health and possible diseases.

Medical specimens for laboratory include a large variety of samples, such as blood, urine, stool, sputum and so on. Such specimens are contained in plastic tubes and sent to the pathology department along with a label or a barcode specifying the patient's name, his unit number and the undergoing test. Once the specimen arrives, the pathologist scans the barcode and the laboratory machines are set to work.

Blood sample is used for a variety of blood tests to measure the physiological and biochemical state of the patient. It is the most important method of uncovering common diseases. It is also an effective way for detecting pregnancy. Blood tests during pregnancy may also help check problems that might affect you and your baby. There are two ways for drawing blood from the human body, venipuncture and finger pricking, depending on the amount of blood needed for the examination.

Urine sample is obtained for clinical urine tests to measure the kidney function and detect possible renal diseases. The common tests include urinalysis (UA) and naked-eye examination for colour, smell and other substances. The UA checks for three things, proteinuria, haematuria and pH value. The protein appears in the urine during kidney diseases, while blood showing up indicates infection and other problems. UA should be taken as a part of a routine check of health, for it's an effective way to find certain diseases in their earlier stages.

Stool sample is collected for an analysis of fecal matter. For example, if you've been having stomach problems, the doctor might order a stool test for you. The test examines your stool for bacteria, a virus, or other germs that might be causing the problem. The tests include a naked eye exam, microbiology tests and chemical tests. The pathologist performs a naked eye exam to check the colour and the texture of the stool, which signal possible diseases of the digestive tracts. Microbiology tests are used to uncover parasitic diseases whereas chemical tests determine the presence of any possible infection.

Sputum, also referred to as phlegm, is a gluey substance that comes up from the lung. It is sent for naked eye exam for its colour and texture and microbiological investigation for any respiratory infection, such as bronchitis, bronchopneumonia or pneumonia.

A medical test is the basis for disease diagnosis, monitoring and further treatment. Accuracy of a medical test depends on correct method of obtaining the sample. Therefore, the procedure should be performed with proper guidance.

🎧 Key Words

laboratory / ləˈbɒrətri / *n.* 实验室

stool / stuːl / *n.* 粪便

sputum / ˈspjuːtəm / *n.* 痰

barcode / ˈbɑːkəʊd / *n.* 条形码

physiological / ˌfɪziəˈlɒdʒɪkl / *adj.* 生理的

biochemical / ˌbaɪəʊˈkemɪkl / *adj.* 生物化学的

pathologist / pəˈθɒlədʒɪst / *n.* 病理医生

prick / prɪk / *v.* 刺，扎

renal / ˈriːnl / *adj.* 肾脏的

urinalysis / ˌjʊərɪˈnælɪsɪs / *n.* 尿分析

proteinuria / ˌprəʊtiːnˈjʊəriə / *n.* 蛋白尿

haematuria / ˌheməˈtjʊəriə / *n.* 血尿

fecal / ˈfiːkl / *adj.* 排泄物的

microbiology / ˌmaɪkrəʊbaɪˈɒlədʒi / *n.* 微生物学

digestive / daɪˈdʒestɪv / *adj.* 消化的

parasitic / ˌpærəˈsɪtɪk / *adj.* 寄生物的

phlegm / flem / *n.* 痰

bronchitis / brɒnˈkaɪtɪs/ *n.* 支气管炎

bronchopneumonia / ˌbrɒnkə(ʊ)njuːˈməʊniə / *n.* 支气管肺炎

pneumonia / njuːˈməʊniə / *n.* 肺炎

Useful Expressions

medical laboratory　医学实验室

naked eye exam　肉眼检测

pH value　pH 值

Exercise

I **Choose the best answer to each question based on the text.**

1. What is the purpose of doing laboratory tests? _____.

　A. To do research on new drugs

　B. To train the medical students

　C. To get to know the patient's condition

2. Which of the following is NOT a possible medical specimen, according to the text? _____.

　A. Drug　　　　　　B. Blood　　　　　　C. Sputum

3. Which way of blood drawing is used when a large amount of blood is needed for tests? _____.

    A. Venipuncture   B. Finger pricking   C. Both A and B

4. Which substance may exist in a patient's urine while he has severe renal diseases? _____.

    A. Blood   B. Protein   C. Salt

5. Which specimen should be tested when a patient suffers from possible respiratory diseases? _____.

    A. Sputum   B. Stool   C. Urine

II Match each medical term in Column A with its explanation in Column B.

Column A		Column B
_____	1. proteinuria	a. the presence of red blood cells in the urine
_____	2. haematuria	b. the invasion of the body by certain bacteria
_____	3. venipuncture	c. the presence of excessive protein in the urine
_____	4. pneumonia	d. puncturing of a vein
_____	5. infection	e. an inflammatory condition of the lung

III Find words or terms in the article to match the following definitions.

1. a doctor who examines the specimen with the help of medical equipment _____

2. a way of drawing blood from the patient's vein for medical examination _____

3. a test which measures the kidney function and detects renal diseases _____

4. a kind of specimen that can be used to investigate respiratory infections _____

IV Critical thinking.

According to the case at the beginning of this unit, what are nursing diagnoses and nursing interventions for the patient?

1. Nursing diagnoses

    • Altered patterns of urinary elimination related to urgency, frequency and pain

    • Altered nutrition related to loss of appetite

2. Nursing interventions

The patient is suggested to have a urine specimen test done immediately. The discomfort associated with a UTI is relieved soon after antibiotic therapy is started. Sitz baths may also help relieve the pain. Avoid catheterization if possible, but it is necessary to maintain an unobstructed flow of urine. Remind the patient to void frequently. Education focuses on preventing the recurrence of a UTI.

Part 4 Supplementary Reading

🎧 Blood Test

Blood test is the most commonly seen laboratory analysis in hospitals around the world, for it provides a full picture of a patient's physiological and biochemical states. Based on the mineral content and organ function it uncovers, the doctor can make a diagnosis and prescribe further treatment. There are three types of blood tests: cellular evaluation, molecular analysis and biochemical analysis.

The complete blood count (CBC), which is also known as full blood count (FBC), is one of the basic cellular analyses and used to detect the cells in a patient's blood. The cells, including white blood cells, red blood cells and platelets, are active members in the bloodstream. Abnormality of any of these three cells indicates potential problems to a patient's health and possible diseases, for example, a high white blood cell indicating an infection, a low red blood cell signaling iron deficiency, a low platelet revealing blood clotting malfunction, etc.

Molecular analysis includes tests of liver function, DNA and sexually transmitted diseases and so on. Take liver function tests as an example. The test shows the state of a patient's liver and whether there are any damage to the liver or some diseases. Liver diseases can be detected in an early stage and thus treatments will follow up.

Biochemical analysis measures the mineral content of a patient's blood, including magnesium, sodium, potassium, glucose, etc. The two most commonly performed analyses are blood glucose measurement for (potential) diabetic patients and measurement for cholesterol levels.

A blood test report is a type of pathology report which is written by a pathologist and contains information about the analysis of the specimen and a diagnosis based on the pathologist's examination. Specifically, a blood test report contains four sections of information: the date of the examination, the patient's personal information (patient's name, age, unit number, etc.), the pathologist's contact information (pathologist's name, the laboratory, contact number, etc.) and details about the specimen (type of test, name of the test items, result of each item, normal range for reference, pathologist's diagnosis, etc.). Here is a pathology report of Complete Blood Count.

St. Jones Hospital **Report for CBC**	Patrick J. Lawrence 16th June 2017 Unit No. 3159762 Dept. of Neurology	

Item	value	Normal Range for reference
WBC	6.6	$(4.3\text{-}10.8) \times 10^9/L$
RBC	4.56	$(4.2\text{-}5.9) \times 10^{12}/L$
Hemoglobin (Hbg)	14.2	120-165 g/L (men); 110-150 g/L (women)
Hematocrit (Hct)	34.2%	45%-52% (men); 37%-48% (women)
mean corpuscular volume (MCV)	79.2	80-94 fL
mean corpuscular hemoglobin (MCH)	26.3	27-32 fL
platelet count	282	$(125\text{-}320) \times 10^9/L$
mean platelet volume (MPV)	10.9	8.8-12.8 fL

Once the test is finished, the blood test report is formed and sent to the ward through hospital intranet. The doctor will make diagnosis and prescribe medications based on the blood results.

Exercise

Choose the best answer to each question based on the text.

1. What is the basic type of cellular analyses? _____.

   A. The Complete Blood Count

   B. DNA test

   C. Biochemical test

2. What is the CBC used to detect? _____.

   A. The liver function

   B. The minerals in a patient's blood

   C. The cells in a patient's blood

3. The test of sexually transmitted diseases belongs to _____ analysis.

   A. cellular   B. molecular   C. biochemical

4. A test of _____ is commonly used to evaluate the condition of diabetic patients.

   A. blood glucose

   B. cholesterol

   C. mineral

5. _____ is responsible of writing a blood test report.

   A. The ward nurse

   B. The pathologist

   C. The doctor

Part 5 Medical Word Elements

1. urin(o)-	尿
urinalysis / ˌjʊərɪˈnælɪsɪs /	尿液分析（法）
urinology / ˌjʊərɪˈnɒədʒi /	泌尿科学
2. patho-	病理
pathology / pəˈθɒlədʒi /	病理学
pathologist / pəˈθɒlədʒɪst /	病理医生
3. -ology	学科
stomatology / ˌstəʊməˈtɒlədʒi /	口腔医学
neurology / ˌnjʊəˈrɒlədʒi /	神经病学
4. -rrhage	出血
haemorrhage / ˈhemərɪdʒ /	（大）出血
hemorrhage / ˈhemərɪdʒ /	（大）出血
5. -uria	尿
hematuria / ˌhiːməˈtjuːrɪə /	血尿
proteinuria / ˌprəʊtiːˈnjʊərɪə /	蛋白尿
6. micro-	小，细微
microbiology / ˌmaɪkrəʊbaɪˈɒlədʒi /	微生物学
microscope / ˈmaɪkrəskəʊp /	显微镜
7. -ium	元素
sodium / ˈsəʊdɪəm /	钠
potassium / pəˈtæsɪəm /	钾
8. dia-	透过
dialysance / daɪˈælɪsəns /	透析率
dialysis / daɪˈælɪsɪs /	透析
9. -lysis	分解，溶解
hemodialysis / ˌhiːmədaɪˈælɪsɪs /	血液透析，肾透析
enzymolysis / ˌenzaɪˈmɒlɪsɪs /	酶解（作用）
10. -itis	炎症
trachitis / trəˈkaɪtɪs /	气管炎
hepatitis / ˌhepəˈtaɪtɪs /	肝炎

（孙韵雪　赵　静）

Medical Imaging

Learning Objectives:

1. *Discussing how to prepare a patient for radiology*
2. *Giving the definition and procedures of CT scan*
3. *Describing the functions and the procedures of B-ultrasonography*
4. *Explaining the types and functions of medical imaging*

Lead-In

Case Study

A middle-aged man came to the emergency room complaining a severe and sudden pain in the abdomen. He presented with high grade fever, nausea, vomiting and watery diarrhoea, sometimes green in colour. On exam, the patient was hypotensive and was looking acutely ill. After receiving some IV fluids, the patient continued to have abdominal pain. The doctor ordered a right upper quadrant ultrasound which showed thickened gall bladder wall of up to 1 cm consistent with cholecystitis.

Part 1 Dialogue

🎧 Preparing a Patient for Radiology

Dr. Peterson, a SHO, is talking about how to preparing a patient for radiology with two nurses, Tina, a ward nurse, and Sarah, a student nurse.

Dr. Peterson: Good morning, let's talk about preparing a patient for radiology. Tina, what about appointment?

Tina: Each patient will receive a call from a nurse at least five days prior to the appointment unless the appointment is made less than five days prior to the scheduled date and time. What will the nurse do during the call, Sarah?

Sarah: During this call, the nurse reviews the patient's medical history and medication list and gives the patient instructions based on the type of procedure that is scheduled.

Dr. Peterson: Well, when should the patient arrive?

Tina: Patients who are undergoing outpatient procedures should arrive 1 hour before their scheduled appointment time and check-in at the radiology front desk.

Sarah: Ok, I remember.

Dr. Peterson: What about the patients who are undergoing a procedure that requires overnight observation?

Tina: Patients should arrive 1.5 hours before their scheduled appointment time and should stop by the admitting office prior to checking in at the radiology front desk.

Sarah: And patients should leave all valuables at home.

Dr. Peterson: Very good. What should the patient do who will receive sedation or anaesthesia during their procedure?

Tina: Patients must have someone available to drive them home and care for them for the next 24 hours.

Sarah: A friend or family member is OK, that is right?

Dr. Peterson: Yes. How long will the procedures that involve sedation?

Tina: Most procedures will last 1 to 2 hours with a 2- to 4-hour recovery period following the procedures.

Sarah: So the patient should expect to be here for at least 3 to 6 hours.

Dr. Peterson: Mm. And NPO (fasting) and medication instructions are very important. Please talk about it.

Tina: Patients who will receive sedation or anaesthesia during the procedure need to be NPO.

Sarah: I know for the patients, no solid food or milk products for 6 hours prior to the procedure and no clear liquids for 2 hours prior to the procedure.

Dr. Peterson: OK. Take all regular medications as scheduled with small sips of water unless otherwise directed. What about medicine for diabetes?

Tina: The diabetic patients take only half dose of evening insulin. What should the diabetic patients do?

Sarah: They should hold morning insulin and oral diabetic medication the day of the procedure.

Dr. Peterson: Yes. Prior to the procedure, what other medications should need to be held?

Tina: There are many anticoagulants, aspirins and non-steroidal anti-inflammatory medications that may need to be held prior to our procedure. Patients should be asked to keep medical team informed of all medications the patient is taking.

Sarah: I understand. Every members of a medical team should know all medications the patient is taking.

Dr. Peterson: All right. If needed, prior to a procedure, our team can review specific medications and plan to manage anticoagulation.

🎧 Key Words

radiology / ˌreɪdɪˈɒlədʒi / n. 放射学

outpatient / ˈaʊtpeɪʃnt / n. 门诊病人

sedation / sɪˈdeɪʃn / n. 镇静；镇静作用

anaesthesia / ˌænəsˈθiːziə / n. 麻醉

fasting / 'fɑːstɪŋ / *n.* 禁食

sip / sɪp / *n.* 抿；小口喝

anticoagulant / ˌæntikəʊˈæɡjulənt / *n.* 抗凝血剂

steroidal / stəˈrɔɪdəl / *adj.* 甾族的，类固醇

anti-inflammatory / ˌænti ɪnˈflæmətri / *adj.* 抗炎的

anticoagulation / ˌæntikəʊˌæɡjuˈleɪʃn / *n.* 抗凝

Useful Expressions

medical imaging　医学影像

medical history　病史；病历

NPO= nil per os = nothing by mouth　禁食

non-steroidal anti-inflammatory medication　非甾体抗炎药

Exercise

I　Read the dialogue again and decide whether the following statements are right or wrong. If there is not enough information to answer "Right" or "Wrong", choose "Doesn't say".

1. During the call, the nurse only gives the patient instructions based on the type of procedure that is scheduled. _____.

　　A. Right　　　　　　B. Wrong　　　　　　C. Doesn't say

2. Patients who are undergoing outpatient procedures should arrive 1 hour before their scheduled appointment time. _____.

　　A. Right　　　　　　B. Wrong　　　　　　C. Doesn't say

3. Patients who will receive injection during the procedure need to be NPO. _____.

　　A. Right　　　　　　B. Wrong　　　　　　C. Doesn't say

4. The diabetic patients should hold morning insulin and oral diabetic medication the day of the procedure. _____.

　　A. Right　　　　　　B. Wrong　　　　　　C. Doesn't say

5. The medical team doesn't need to know all medications the patient is taking. _____.

　　A. Right　　　　　　B. Wrong　　　　　　C. Doesn't say

II　Discussion.

How to prepare a patient for radiology?

Part 2　Short Passage

🎧 CT Scan

A CT scan, also known as computed tomography scan, makes use of computer-processed combinations of many X-ray measurements taken from different angles to produce cross-sectional (tomographic) images (virtual "slices") of specific areas of a scanned object, allowing the user to see inside the object without cutting. Other terms include computed axial tomography (CAT scan) and computer aided tomography.

The term "computed tomography" (CT) is often used to refer to X-ray CT. Medical imaging is the most common application of X-ray CT. Its cross-sectional images are used for diagnostic and therapeutic purposes in various medical disciplines. CT produces data that can be manipulated in order to demonstrate various bodily structures based on their ability to absorb the X-ray beam.

Procedures for computerized axial tomography (CAT scan):

1. Explain the purpose of the procedure to the patient.

2. Identify allergies to shellfish or iodine.

3. Obtain the permit.

4. Place the patient on NPO as dye could cause nausea.

5. Administer the medication preprocedure if ordered.

6. Take the patient on a gurney to the X-ray department.

7. Explain equipment and need for patient's head to be placed in a rubber cap.

8. Explain that a warm, flushed feeling or nausea could occur during test.

9. Instruct the patient to lie very still during the procedure.

10. Return the patient to his/her room.

11. Provide diet and forced fluids of 3000 mL as ordered.

12. Medicate the headache if needed.

There are several advantages that CT has over traditional 2D medical radiography. First, CT completely eliminates the superimposition of images of structures outside the area of interest. Second, because of the inherent high-contrast resolution of CT, differences between tissues that differ on physical density by less than 1% can be distinguished. Finally, data from a single CT imaging procedure consisting of either multiple contiguous or one helical scan can be viewed as images in the axial, coronal, or sagittal planes, depending on the diagnostic task.

🎧 Key Words

scan / skæn / n./v. 扫描

tomography / tə'mɒgrəfi / n. X 线断层摄影术

cross-sectional / krɒs'sekʃənl / adj. 截面的，断面的

virtual / 'vɜːtʃuəl / adj. 虚拟的

therapeutic / ˌθerə'pjuːtɪk / adj. 治疗的

shellfish / 'ʃelfɪʃ / n. 甲壳类动物

iodine / 'aɪədiːn / n. 碘

gurney / 'gɜːni / n.（移动病人用的）轮床

superimposition / ˌsuːpəˌɪmpə'zɪʃn / n. 叠印；重加

inherent / ɪn'hɪərənt / adj. 固有的；内在的

contrast / 'kɒntrɑːst / n. 对比

resolution / ˌrezə'luːʃn / n. 分辨率

contiguous / kən'tɪgjuəs / adj. 连续的；邻近的

helical / 'helɪkl / adj. 螺旋形的

coronal / kə'rəʊnl / adj. 冠状的

sagittal / 'sædʒɪtl / adj. 矢状的；箭头形的

Useful Expressions

computed tomography (CT) scan　计算机断层扫描

computed axial tomography (CAT scan)(= computerized axial tomography)　计算机轴向断层成像

computer aided tomography　计算机辅助断层扫描

X-ray CT　X 射线 CT

high-contrast resolution　高对比度分辨率

Exercise

I Choose the best answer to each question based on the text.

1. A CT scan makes use of computer-processed combinations of many X-ray measurements to produce _____.

   A. cross-sectional images　　B. helical images　　C. coronal images

2. A CT scan can _____.

   A. only be taken from the same angle

   B. produce virtual "slices" of specific areas of a scanned object

   C. allow the user to see the cutting inside the object

3. What does "discipline" in Paragraph 2 mean? _____.

   A. A system of rules of conduct or method of practice

   B. A branch of knowledge

   C. Training to improve strength or self-control

4. Which statement is incorrect? _____.

   A. CT images are used for diagnostic and therapeutic purposes

   B. CT data demonstrate various bodily structures based on their ability to absorb the X-ray beam

   C. CT has several advantages over traditional 3D medical radiography

5. Differences between tissues that differ in physical density by less than 1% can be distinguished because of _____.

   A. the acquired low-contrast resolution of CT

   B. the inherent high-contrast resolution of CT

   C. the acquired high-contrast revolution of CT

II Read the passage again and put the following extracts in the correct order.

☐ **A** Instruct the patient to lie very still during the procedure.

☐ **B** Place the patient on NPO as dye could cause nausea.

☐ **C** Administer the medication preprocedure if ordered.

☐ **D** Place the patient's head in a rubber cap.

☐ **E** Identify allergies to shellfish or iodine.

☐ **F** Provide diet and forced fluids to 3000 mL as ordered.

☐ **G** Take the patient on a gurney to the X-ray department.

🎧 Ultrasonography

Ultrasonography is a form of body imaging using sound waves to facilitate making a medical diagnosis. A skilled ultrasound technician is able to see inside the body using ultrasonography to answer questions that may be asked by the medical practitioner caring for the patient. In B-ultrasonography, a two-dimensional image can be viewed on screen, more commonly known as 2D mode now.

Usually, a radiologist will oversee the ultrasound test and report on the results, but other types of physicians may also use ultrasound as a diagnostic tool. For example, obstetricians use ultrasound to assess the fetus during pregnancy. Surgeons and emergency physicians use ultrasound at the bedside to assess abdominal pain or other concerns.

Before the exam, the patient will change into a hospital gown. He will most likely be lying down on a table with a section of his body exposed for the test. An ultrasound technician, called a sonographer, will apply a special lubricating gel to the patient's skin. This prevents friction so they can rub the ultrasound transducer on the patient's skin. The transducer has a similar appearance to a microphone. The gel also helps transmit the sound waves. The transducer sends high-frequency sound waves through a patient's body. The waves echo as they hit a dense object, such as an organ or bone. Those echoes are then reflected back into a computer. The sound waves are at too high of a pitch for the human ear to hear. They form a picture that can be interpreted by the doctor. Depending on the area being examined, the patient may need to change positions so the technician can have better access. After the procedure, the gel will be cleaned off of the skin. The whole procedure typically lasts less than 30 minutes, depending on the area being examined. A patient will be free to go about his normal activities after the procedure has finished.

The physics of sound can place limits on the test. The quality of the picture depends on many factors. Sound waves cannot penetrate deeply, and an obese patient may be imaged poorly. Ultrasound does poorly when gas is present between the probe and the target organ. Should the intestine be distended with bowel gas, organs behind it may not be easily seen. Similarly, ultrasound works poorly in the chest, where the lungs are filled with air. Ultrasound does not penetrate bone easily. The accuracy of the test is very much operator-dependent. This means that the key to a good test is the ultrasound technician.

Ultrasound can be enhanced by using Doppler technology which can measure whether an object is moving towards or away from the probe. This can allow the technician to measure blood flow in organs such as the heart or livers, or within specific blood vessels.

🎧 Key Words

ultrasonography / ˌʌltrəsəˈnɒgrəfi / *n.* 超声波检查法

ultrasound / ˈʌltrəsaʊnd / *n.* 超声；超声波

dimensional / dɪˈmenʃənl / *adj.* 空间的，维度的

obstetrician / ˌɒbstəˈtrɪʃn / *n.* 产科医生

sonographer / ˈsɒnəgrɑːfə / *n.* 超声波检验师

lubricating / ˈluːbrɪkeɪtɪŋ/ *adj.* 润滑的

gel / dʒel / *n.* 凝胶

transducer / trænzˈdjuːsə / *n.* 传感器

echo / ˈekəʊ / *vi.* 发出回音

dense / dens / *adj.* 密实的

penetrate / ˈpenətreɪt / *v.* 穿透

intestine / ɪnˈtestɪn / *n.* 肠

Doppler / ˈdɒplə / *adj.* 多普勒效应的

Useful Expressions

B-ultrasonography   B 超

two-dimensional image   二维图像

target organ   目标器官

Doppler technology   多普勒技术

Exercise

Ⅰ Choose the best answer to each question based on the text.

1. B-ultrasonography can produce a _____ image.

   A. two-dimensional   B. three-dimensional   C. four-dimensional

2. Which of the following is NOT the application of ultrasonography? _____.

   A. To assess the fetus by obstetricians

   B. To assess tooth decay by dentists

   C. To assess abdominal pain by surgeons

3. To avoid friction, _____ is used.

   A. transducer   B. probe   C. gel

4. The quality of the picture depends on many factors, except _____.

   A. the doctor's mood

   B. the skill of the operator

   C. gas in the target organ

5. In order to measure blood flow in the heart, _____ technology is applied.

   A. Modern   B. Doppler   C. Pine

Ⅱ Match each medical term in Column A with its explanation in Column B.

	Column A	Column B
_____	1. dimensional	a. an electrical device that converts one form of energy into another
_____	2. ultrasound	b. a diagnostic medical professional
_____	3. sonographer	c. very high frequency sound

| | 4. lubricating | d. of making slippery or smooth |
| | 5. transducer | e. of or relating to magnitude or extent |

Ⅲ Find words or terms in the article to match the following definitions.

1. using the reflections of high-frequency sound waves to construct an image of a body organ

_____

2. a doctor who is trained in radiology _____

3. a physician specializing in obstetrics _____

4. the part of the alimentary canal between the stomach and the anus _____

Ⅳ Critical thinking.

According to the case at the beginning of this unit, what are nursing diagnoses and nursing interventions for the patient?

1. Nursing diagnoses

- Fluid volume deficit related to nausea, vomiting and diarrhoea
- Alteration in nutrition: less than body requirements related to nausea and vomiting and diarrhoea secondary to cholecystitis
- Pain related to inflammation of the gallbladder

2. Nursing interventions

Analgesics are administered to provide relief from pain. The nurse enforces the patient's NOP (Nothing by Mouth) status. An intravenous line is started for replacement of fluids and electrolytes lost from vomiting and diarrhoea. The IV line is also used for the administration of antibiotics. The patient's intake and output are closely monitored, noting the colour and amount of the urine and stool. Education about dietary restriction of fatty, high-cholesterol and spicy food are given for the patient.

Part 4 Supplementary Reading

🎧 Medical Imaging

Medical imaging is a discipline within the medical field which involves the use of technology to take images of the inside of the human body. These images are used in diagnostics as teaching tools, and in routine health care for a variety of conditions. Medical imaging is sometimes referred to as diagnostic imaging, because it is frequently used to help doctors arrive at a diagnosis, and there are a number of different types of technology used in imaging.

The goal of imaging is to provide a picture of the inside of the body in a way which is as non-invasive as possible. An imaging study can be used to identify unusual things inside the body, such as broken bones, tumours, leaking blood vessels, and so forth. One of the most famous types of diagnostic imaging is the X-ray, which uses radiation to take a static image of a specific area of the body.

In addition to X-rays and related computed tomography (CT) technology, it is also possible to use ultrasound to look inside the body by bouncing sound waves from the body cavity to make a picture, and to utilize magnetic resonance imaging to agitate the cells to get a picture of the body. Medical imaging can also produce dynamic images, such as scans of brain activity or pictures of the heart in motion which can be used to look for diagnostic issues which would not appear in a static image. More invasive techniques involve the insertion of a camera into the body to take video of an area of interest.

Some imaging studies simply require a capture of an image, while others involve the introduction of a contrast material to the body. Contrast materials are swallowed or injected, and they are designed to be highly visible in the picture, allowing a doctor to follow their progress through the body. A barium swallow, for example, may be used in an X-ray of the digestive tract to look for ulcers and perforations, while radioactive contrasts may be injected to look for signs of thyroid cancer.

New technology for medical imaging is being developed all the time, including machines which are less invasive and technology which reduces the need for radioactive materials and other harmful substances in imaging. Molecular imaging is used in nuclear medicine and a variety of methods are used to visualize biological processes taking place in the cells of organisms. Small amounts of radioactive markers, called radiopharmaceuticals, are used for molecular imaging. Molecular imaging provides detailed information of the biological processes taking place in the body at cellular and molecular levels and can indicate disease in its earliest stages.

Other types of medical imaging are magnetic resonance imaging (MRI) and ultrasound imaging. Unlike conventional X-ray, CT and molecular imaging, MRI and ultrasound operate without ionizing radiation. MRI uses strong magnetic fields, which produce unknown irreversible biological effects in humans. Diagnostic ultrasound systems use high-frequency sound waves to produce images of soft tissue and internal body organs.

Exercise

Choose the best answer to each question based on the text.
1. Medical images can be used in _____.

   A. diagnostics   B. routine health care   C. both A and B
2. X-ray uses radiation to take a (n) _____ image of a specific area of the body.

   A. static   B. dynamic   C. invasive
3. A barium swallow may be used in an X-ray of the _____ to look for ulcers.

   A. respiratory tract   B. intestinal tract   C. digestive tract
4. New technology for medical imaging needs _____.

   A. fewer harmful substances

   B. fewer radioactive materials

C. both A and B

5. How many types of medical imaging technology are referred to in this article? _____.

   A. 2   B. 5   C. 6

Part 5 Medical Word Elements

1. ultra-	超
ultrasonics / ˌʌltrəˈsɒnɪks /	超声学
ultramicroscopic / ˌʌltrəˌmaɪkrəˈskɒpɪk /	超显微镜的
2. -scope	镜
laparoscope / ˈlæpərəskəup /	腹腔镜
enteroscope / ˈentərəskəup /	肠镜
3. -scopy	检查法
gastroscopy / gæsˈtrɒskəpi /	胃镜检查〔法〕
colonoscopy / ˌkəulənəˈskɒpi /	结肠镜检查（法）
4. -graph	描记器，照相
angiograph / ændʒiˈəugræf /	血管造影照片
cardiograph / ˈkɑːdiəgrɑːf /	心动描记器；心电图
5. -graphy	书写，记录，造影术
angiography / ændʒɪˈɒgrəfi /	血管造影术
radiography / ˌreɪdiˈɒgrəfi /	X 线摄影（术）
6. chrom(o)-	色
chromosome / ˈkrəuməsəum /	染色体
chromoscopy / krəuˈmɒskəpi /	染色检查
7. thym(o)-	胸腺
thymitis / θaɪˈmaɪtɪs /	胸腺炎
thymoma / θaɪˈməumə /	胸腺瘤
8. lith(o)-	结石
lithogenic / ˌlɪθəˈdʒenɪk /	促结石形成的
lithoclastic / ˌlɪθəuˈklæstɪk /	碎石的
9. sten(o)-	狭窄
stenosis / stɪˈnəusɪs /	狭窄病
stenocephaly / ˌstenəˈsefəli /	头狭窄

（钱　超　罗晓冰）

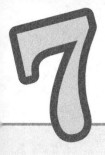

Caring for a Preoperative Patient

Learning Objectives:

1. *Discussing the role of the practitioner in preparing a patient for his/her operation*
2. *Describing the content of preoperative nursing*
3. *Discussing different types of enema administration*
4. *Explaining the significance of informed consent*

Lead-In

Case Study

Michelle Smits, a 28-year-old, had been bleeding when defecating for two weeks. Through a diagnostic colonoscopy—the examination of bowel through an endoscope, three polyps were discovered in her colon. Michelle was booked for elective bowel surgery tomorrow. She was feeling nervous about the operation and had some trouble falling asleep. What preoperative instruction should the nurse give to the patient?

Part 1 Dialogue

🎧 Preoperative Check

Alexandra, the ward nurse, prepares Mr. Dawson for his operation by telling him about the preoperative routine in the ward.

Alexandra: Good afternoon, Mr. Dawson. I'm your charge nurse, Alexandra. I will be looking after you today. Have you settled in yet?

Mr. Dawson: Good afternoon, Alexandra. Yes, I just have to wait for the operation now, don't I?

Alexandra: Yes, I'm going to look at the operation list when it comes out later today so I can tell you where you are on the list. I just need to go through some preoperative things with you. Is that OK?

Mr. Dawson: Yeah, that's fine.

Alexandra: Right, let me see. First, I'll check your consent form. Is that your signature?

Mr. Dawson: Yes, I signed it in the doctor's surgery before I came to the hospital.

Alexandra: Good, you'll also need to shower with this antiseptic wash. Here's a sachet of the wash for you. Just wash all over using the antiseptic wash as you would with soap.

Mr. Dawson: All right. I'll do that tonight before I go to bed.

Alexandra: Great. We'll prepare you by shaving and cleaning your abdomen tomorrow morning.

Mr. Dawson: I see.

Alexandra: I'm going to order you clear fluids for today. That means you'll just be on liquids today. Then you'll eat nothing by mouth after midnight.

Mr. Dawson: Oh yes. That means I won't be able to eat or drink anything after midnight, will I?

Alexandra: No, you won't. The reason for this is that when you have an anaesthetic, your muscles relax. If you have anything in your stomach it could rise up into your throat and you might inhale it. It's very dangerous.

Mr. Dawson: OK. I see. I certainly don't want that to happen.

Alexandra: In the early morning you'll have an enema so that when the surgeon operates, there is less chance of contamination from the bowel contents.

Mr. Dawson: I got it.

Alexandra: Now I will ask you some questions. If you don't understand, I will explain them to you.

Mr. Dawson: Of course.

Alexandra: Have you been allergic to any medication or foods?

Mr. Dawson: Let me see. Oh, I'm allergic to seafood.

Alexandra: Your blood type is A, right?

Mr. Dawson: Yes.

Alexandra: Do you sleep well? If you are suffering from insomnia, the doctor will give you some sleeping pills.

Mr. Dawson: Not very well. Please give me some, thank you.

Alexandra: You look worried. Do you have any concerns?

Mr. Dawson: My operation is the keyhole surgery, right? What's that?

Alexandra: That's right. Um, keyhole surgery is also called minimally invasive surgery because it's performed with the use of a laparoscope, using small incisions or surgical cuts. You'll probably have three to four puncture sites. There are just small holes made near your navel. And you will have a small dressing covering the holes made during surgery. It's just a light covering to keep area clean until it heals.

Mr. Dawson: Ah-ha. I got it.

Alexandra: Well, tomorrow morning I will take your vital signs including your body temperature, blood pressure and heart rate. So have a good rest.

Mr. Dawson: OK, thank you.

🎧 Key Words

enema / ˈenəmə / n. 灌肠法；灌肠剂

cholecystectomy / ˌkɒlɪsɪsˈtektəmi / n. 胆囊切除术

shave / ʃeɪv / v. 剃须，剃毛

anaesthetic / ˌænəsˈθetɪk / n. 麻醉剂，麻药

insomnia / ɪnˈsɒmnɪə / *n.* 失眠症，失眠　　　　navel / ˈneɪvl / *n.* 肚脐
laparoscope / ˈlæpərəskəʊp / *n.* 腹腔镜

Useful Expressions

settle in 安顿下来　　　　　　　　　　　　be allergic to 对……过敏
consent form 知情同意书

Exercise

I　**Read the dialogue again and decide whether the following statements are right or wrong. If there is not enough information to answer "Right" or "Wrong", choose "Doesn't say".**

1. The nurse is talking with Mr. Dawson about preoperative preparations. _____.
   A. Right　　　　　　B. Wrong　　　　　　C. Doesn't say
2. Mr. Dawson should take a bath tomorrow morning. _____.
   A. Right　　　　　　B. Wrong　　　　　　C. Doesn't say
3. Mr. Dawson can drink some water but can NOT eat food tonight. _____.
   A. Right　　　　　　B. Wrong　　　　　　C. Doesn't say
4. Anxiety can raise the blood pressure. _____.
   A. Right　　　　　　B. Wrong　　　　　　C. Doesn't say
5. Mr. Dawson must take sleeping pills before going to bed. _____.
   A. Right　　　　　　B. Wrong　　　　　　C. Doesn't say

II　**Discussion.**

What preparations should Mr. Dawson make for his abdominal surgery?

Part 2　Short Passage

🎧 Enema Administration

An enema administration is the injection of fluid into the lower bowel by way of the rectum. The most frequent use of an enema is to relieve constipation or for bowel cleansing before a medical examination or procedure. The process helps push waste out of the rectum when you cannot do so on your own. Enemas are available for purchase at pharmacies for home use, but you should ask a doctor or nurse for specific instructions to avoid injury.

Types of enemas

There are several common types of enemas. The purpose of a cleansing enema is to gently flush out the colon. It may be recommended prior to a colonoscopy or other medical examination. Constipation, fatigue, headaches, and backaches may be relieved by a cleansing enema. During a cleansing enema, a water-based solution with a small concentration of stool softener, baking soda, or apple cider vinegar is used to stimulate the movement of the large intestine. A cleansing enema should stimulate the bowels to quickly expel both the solution and any impacted fecal matter. A retention enema also stimulates the bowels, but the solution is intended to be "held" in the body for 15 minutes or more.

Procedures for an enema

1. Position: Raise bed to a high position and lay down side rails. Place a bed protector under the patient. Place the patient on the left side in a Sim's position.

2. Preparation: Fill water container with 750 to 1000 mL of lukewarm solution. Allow solution to run through the tubing so that air was removed. Lubricate the tip of the tubing with water-soluble lubricant.

3. Implementation: Gently insert the tubing 3-4 inches into the patients' rectum, past the external and internal sphincters. Raise the water container to a maximum height of 18 inches to allow solution to flow slowly. Hold the tubing in place in the patients' rectum at all times. Keep a bedpan nearby.

4. Follow-up: After the solution was instilled, gently remove the tubing. Instruct patient to hold solution for 10-15 minutes. Elevate the head of the bed so that the patient could assume a squatting position on the bedpan or be assisted to bathroom. Remove and cover bedpan.

5. Ending: Clean all the equipment and replace them in the bathroom or an appropriate location. Wash hands.

After an enema

Some people find that they have several additional bowel movements in the hours after an enema. For this reason, they plan to stay home for the rest of the day after an enema is administered. But for the most part, they may carry on with their regular routine after the enema process is complete. Improper administration of an enema can cause electrolyte imbalance (with repeated enemas) or ruptures to the bowel or rectal tissues resulting in internal bleeding. However, these occurrences are rare in healthy, sober adults. Call physician immediately regarding any adverse effects.

🎧 Key Words

rectum / ˈrektəm / n. 直肠
colonoscopy / ˌkɒləˈnɒskəpi / n. 结肠镜检查术
constipation / ˌkɒnstɪˈpeɪʃn / n. 便秘

electrolyte / ɪˈlektrəlaɪt / n. 电解质
rupture / ˈrʌptʃə(r)/ n. （血管、膀胱等的）破裂

Useful Expressions

be recommended to   被推荐给……
cleansing enema   清洁灌肠

retention enema   保留灌肠

Exercise

I Choose the best answer to each question based on the text.

1. An enema administration begins in the _____.

   A. colon   B. lower bowel   C. rectum

2. Which of the following is NOT the aim of cleansing enema? _____.

   A. To relieve constipation

   B. To clean the colon

   C. To lose weight

3. When choosing a retention enema, you are expected to keep the solution in the body _____.

   A. for 15 minutes   B. for a short time   C. before taking a shower

4. Which of the following statements is NOT correct? _____.

   A. Equipment used should been sterilized

   B. Place the patient on a left-sided position

   C. Insert the tubing more than 4 inches into the rectum

5. After an enema administration, _____ may occur.

   A. headache   B. internal bleeding   C. fatigue

II Read the passage again and put the following extracts in the correct order.

   ☐ **A** Have a lubricant on the tubing.

   ☐ **B** Raise the water container.

   ☐ **C** Place the patient in a Sims' position.

   ☐ **D** Wash hands.

   ☐ **E** Hold the tubing in the patient's rectum.

   ☐ **F** Elevate the head of the bed.

   ☐ **G** Prepare the enema solution.

Part 3 Text

🎧 Preoperative Nursing

Good preparation of surgical patients improves their experience of surgery and anaesthesia and leads to positive outcomes. Nurses play an important role in patient preparation because of their understanding of the perioperative environment and their ability to assess the individual needs of a patient for what is likely to be one of the most significant events of their life.

Preoperative education

Communication with preoperative patients is one of the essential skills that nurses must develop. Research has long shown that informed patients are better prepared for surgery, therefore experience the best outcomes from surgery and anaesthesia, and recover faster. Nurses can employ various teaching strategies to maximize patient education, such as humorous teaching strategies and information leaflets. Preoperative instructions for all patients are summarized as the following:

The need for preoperative tests will be illustrated by nurses to patients, such as laboratory tests, X-ray. If required, they may be asked for bowel preparation. Skin preparations are needed, including the operative area and the preoperative bath. According to the order, nurse should discuss the preoperative medication with patients. Individual therapies ordered by the physician are explained to patients, and at the same time, the visits by the anesthetist are discussed. The requirements of restricted food and oral liquid at least 8 hours before surgery are explained to patients and related postoperative exercises are taught such as deep-breathing and coughing exercises, leg exercises, etc. Patients should be told to remove jewelry, make-up, and all prostheses before surgery.

Preoperative care

Preoperative assessment includes collecting and reviewing specific client data to determine the client's needs. Physical, psychological and social needs are determined during assessment. Preoperatively, the nurse performs a brief but complete physical assessment, paying particular attention to physiological systems that could affect the client's response to anaesthesia or surgery. Physiological assessment looks at areas such as oxygenation, nutrition, elimination, activity and rest, protection, the senses, fluids and electrolytes, neurological and endocrine function. Assessment of the patient's psychosocial needs involves the patient's self-concept, role function and interdependence. Some common nursing diagnoses for preoperative patients are anxiety and deficient knowledge. Nursing planning should involve the patient and support people. Goals for preoperative patients are to be physically, mentally, and emotionally prepared for surgery.

Preoperative examinations

Preoperative patients routinely undergo several examinations or tests. A full blood count (FBC) is carried out to exclude conditions such as anaemia. Patients usually have their blood cross-matched before major procedures, in case blood transfusion is required later, or if the risk is deemed to be small, then their blood is just grouped and saved. Patients undergoing minor procedures, such as day surgery patients, normally have their blood grouped and saved, but not cross-matched. Measuring blood urea and electrolyte levels help to exclude organ disease, for example, diabetes or renal disease.

Effective patient education and preoperative assessment help to prepare the patient effectively for their surgery and anaesthesia. Nurses can act as the patient's advocate and communicate relevant information to the rest of the perioperative team, helping to provide continuity of care.

🎧 Key Words

perioperative / ˌperɪˈɒpərətɪv/ adj. 围术期的　　leaflet / ˈliːflət / n. 传单，散页印刷品

bowel / ˈbaʊəl / n. 肠

order / ˈɔːdə(r)/ n. 医嘱；规定

prosthesis / prɒsˈθiːsɪs / n. 假体（复数 prostheses）

nutrition / njuˈtrɪʃn / n. 营养

elimination / ɪˌlɪmɪˈneɪʃn / n. 排泄

neurological / ˌnjʊərəˈlɒdʒɪkl / adj. 神经系统的

endocrine / ˈendəʊkraɪn / adj. 内分泌的；激素的

anaemia / əˈniːmiə / n. 贫血（症）

diabetes / ˌdaɪəˈbiːtiːz / n. 糖尿病

Useful Expressions

full blood count (FBC)　全血计数

cross-match　交叉配血

deep-breathing　深呼吸

self-concept　自我概念

Exercise

I　Choose the best answer to each question based on the text.

1. The following are effective ways to communicate with the patient except for _____.

　　A. using humorous teaching strategies

　　B. using information leaflets

　　C. holding a competition

2. Preoperative instructions should include _____.

　　A. nothing by mouth at least 8 hours before surgery

　　B. taking a bath after surgery

　　C. wearing prostheses before surgery

3. Which of the following is NOT the area concerned with physiological assessment? _____.

　　A. Nutrition　　　　　　　B. Sleep　　　　C. Self-esteem

4. A 36-year-old woman has anaemia. Which type of preoperative test should she properly undergo?_____.

　　A. Blood cross-match　　　　B. FBC　　　C. Blood urea nitrogen test

5. Preoperative assessment is made to determine the _____ needs of surgical patients.

　　A. physical, social and psychological

　　B. physical, mental and spiritual

　　C. physical, mental and ideological

II　Match each medical term in Column A with its explanation in Column B

	Column A	Column B
_____	1. anaemia	a. a vague unpleasant emotion
_____	2. anxiety	b. loss of bodily sensation with or without loss of consciousness
_____	3. anaesthesia	c. a deficiency of red blood cells
_____	4. oxygenation	d. a solution that conducts electricity
_____	5. electrolytes	e. the process of providing or treating with oxygen

III Find words or terms in the article to match the following definitions.

1. the bodily process of deep inhalation and exhalation _____

2. the activity of conveying information _____

3. to test the compatibility of (a donor's and recipient's blood) by checking that the red cells of each do not agglutinate in the other's serum _____

4. the act of judging a person or situation or event _____

IV Critical thinking.

According to the case at the beginning of this unit, what are nursing diagnoses and nursing interventions for the patient?

1. Nursing diagnoses

   - Anxiety related to general perception about the surgery
   - Risk for infection related to the surgical procedure
   - Risk for fluid volume deficit related to loss of blood and the drainage

2. Nursing interventions

Patient undergoing traditional abdominal surgery requires preoperative teaching. Patient must be taught ways of preventing postoperative complications. The nurse teaches the patient how to use an incentive spirometer. The patient is also instructed to turn, cough, and take deep breaths after the surgery. Many patients are now being placed on patient-controlled analgesia (PCA). The nurse needs to instruct the patient on how to operate the machine.

Part 4 Supplementary Reading

🎧 Informed Consent

Informed consent is a process of getting permission before conducting a health care intervention on a person, or of disclosing personal information. The key to preserving the dignity and autonomy of the patient is informed consent. A health care provider may ask a patient to consent to receive a medical or surgical treatment before providing it, or a clinical researcher may ask a research participant before enrolling that person into a clinical trial to have the rights of understanding the risks involved.

Informed consent is collected according to guidelines from the fields of medical ethics and research ethics. An informed consent can be said to have been given based upon a clear appreciation and understanding of the facts, implications, and consequences of an action. Adequate informed consent is rooted in respecting a person's dignity. To give informed consent, the individual concerned must have adequate reasoning faculties and be in possession of all relevant facts.

Impairments of reasoning and judgement that may prevent informed consent include basic intellectual or emotional immaturity, high levels of stress such as posttraumatic stress disorder (PTSD) or a severe intellectual disability, severe mental disorder, intoxication, severe sleep deprivation,

Alzheimer's disease, or being in a coma.

Obtaining informed consent is not always required. If an individual is considered unable to give informed consent, another person is generally authorized to give consent on his behalf, e.g., parents or legal guardians of a child (though in this circumstance the child may be required to provide informed assent) and conservators for the mentally disordered. Consent can also be assumed through the doctrine of implied consent, e.g., when an unconscious person will die without immediate medical treatment. In cases where an individual is provided insufficient information to form a reasoned decision, serious ethical issues arise. Such cases in a clinical trial in medical research are anticipated and prevented by an ethic committee or Institutional Review Board. Finally, for an individual to give valid informed consent, three components must be present: disclosure, capacity and voluntariness.

Exercise

Choose the best answer to each question based on the text.

1. Informed consent can be used in _____.

    A. hospital   B. research institute   C. both A and B

2. Which of the statements is NOT true according to the passage? _____.

    A. Informed consent is a must under almost any circumstance

    B. Informed consent must be signed in person

    C. A person's dignity is respected through informed consent

3. The informed consent should be signed before _____.

    A. medical treatment   B. hospitalization   C. hospital discharge

4. Implied consent will be assumed if the patient is _____.

    A. unconscious and dying without immediate medical treatment

    B. a newborn

    C. suffering from insomnia

5. A valid informed consent has components except _____.

    A. secret   B. capacity   C. willingness

Part 5 Medical Word Elements

1. pre-   在前

    premedication / ˌpriːˌmedɪˈkeɪʃn /   术前用药

    preoperative / priːˈɒpərətɪv /   术前的

2. varic(o)-   静脉曲张

    varicosis / ˌværɪˈkəʊsɪs /   静脉曲张病

    varicotomy / ˌværɪˈkɒtəmi /   曲张静脉切除术

3. hemat(o)- ; hem(o)-　　　　　　　　　　　血
　　hematocyte / ˈhiːmətəʊsaɪt /　　　　　血细胞
　　hemoglobin / ˌhiːməˈɡləʊbɪn /　　　　血红蛋白
4. -emia; -aemia　　　　　　　　　　　　　血症
　　anaemia / əˈniːmiə /　　　　　　　　　贫血
　　hyperglycemia / ˈhaɪpəɡlaɪˈsiːmiə /　　高血糖
5. anti-　　　　　　　　　　　　　　　　　对抗
　　antibody / ˈæntibɒdi /　　　　　　　　抗体
　　antiseptic / ˌæntiˈseptɪk /　　　　　　抗菌剂
6. hyper-　　　　　　　　　　　　　　　　高
　　hyperlipidemia / ˈhaɪpəˌlɪpɪˈdiːmiə /　高血脂症
　　hypertension / ˌhaɪpəˈtenʃn /　　　　　高血压
7. hypo-　　　　　　　　　　　　　　　　低
　　hypoglycemia / ˌhaɪpəʊɡlaɪˈsiːmiə /　　低血糖
　　hypotension / ˌhaɪpəʊˈtenʃən /　　　　低血压
8. end(o)-　　　　　　　　　　　　　　　　内
　　endocarditis / ˌendəʊkɑːˈdaɪtɪs /　　　心内膜炎
　　endocrine / ˈendəʊkrɪn /　　　　　　　内分泌
9. exo-　　　　　　　　　　　　　　　　　外
　　exotoxin / ˌeksəʊˈtɒksɪn /　　　　　　外毒素
　　exocrine / ˈeksəʊkraɪn /　　　　　　　外分泌

（张佳媛　赵　静）

Caring for a Postoperative Patient

Learning Objectives:

1. *Explaining a postoperative pain*
2. *Describing urinary catheterization and its procedures*
3. *Explaining the process of postoperative nursing*
4. *Describing pain scales*

Lead-In

Case Study

Roli Douglas awoke from a surgery of right shoulder arthroscopy three hours ago. He was started on some IV antibiotics in the left arm and the wound was dressed with non-adhesive dressing. Mr. Douglas complained to the nurse that he was in a lot of pain and he felt dizzy at the moment. He also got a sore throat and thirsty. The nurse took his observations, Temperature: 36.2 ℃, Pulse: 75, Respiration: 18. The IV cannula didn't hurt and the wound was clean and dry.

Part 1 Dialogue

🎧 Explaining a Postoperative Pain

Georgia, a ward nurse, is talking to Roli, a patient after an operation.

Georgia: Hello, Roli. I'll just do some more obs. and see how you're doing.

Roli:　　OK.

Georgia: Are you quite awake after the operation?

Roli:　　Yeah, I'm awake now, um, but I still feel a bit groggy.

Georgia: That's because you've had an anaesthetic. You'll feel better soon.

Roli:　　Thanks. I feel like I'd be sick if I ate anything.

Georgia: Mm, nausea is sometimes a reaction to postoperative pain. I'll keep an eye on that. How's the pain level?

Roli:　　Oh, I'm in bad pain, and everything hurts.

Georgia: That's quite normal. Postoperative pain is an acute pain, and with the correct management it will decrease over a few days or so after the operation, depending on the patient's individual pain tolerance.

Roli： I hope so.

Georgia: Some patients have a high tolerance for pain and some have a low tolerance for pain. Can you rate the pain for me? On a scale of zero to ten, zero is when you feel no pain and ten is when you feel the worst pain that you can imagine. What's the pain like now?

Roli: It's around six.

Georgia: And when you move a bit?

Roli: It gets worse. Seven, at least.

Georgia: I see. Patients who've had an abdominal surgery are often in quite a bit of discomfort. I'll go to get you some medicine for the pain. Analgesics act on different sites of the body and are therefore useful for the various postoperative pains. After you've had the medicine, you might feel like playing one of our video games. Playing games always takes your mind off feeling uncomfortable. Are you warm enough now?

Roli: Um, I'm still feeling cold. Is that normal?

Georgia: Yeah, It's OK. It's called hypothermia. It happens sometimes if the operation takes a long time. I'll get you an extra blanket to help warm you up, because being warm helps the pain as well.

Roli: Good, thanks a lot. And my throat feels really sore. It's hard to swallow.

Georgia: Don't worry, that's normal. It's just caused by the tube they put down your throat during surgery. I'll get some ice chips to suck soon.

Roli: Good, thanks a lot.

🎧 Key Words

groggy / 'grɒgi / *adj.* 无力的；头昏眼花的

nausea / 'nɔ:ziə / *n.* 作呕；恶心

tolerance / 'tɒlərəns / *n.* 忍耐力

abdominal / æb'dɒmɪnl / *adj.* 腹部的

analgesic / ˌænəl'dʒi:zɪk / *n.* 镇痛药

Useful Expressions

obs.=observations　观察

postoperative pain　术后疼痛

pain tolerance　疼痛耐受度

keep an eye on　密切注意……

act on　对……起作用

Exercise

I Read the dialogue again and decide whether the following statements are right or wrong. If there is not enough information to answer "Right" or "Wrong", choose "Doesn't say".

1. The patient's blood pressure is normal. _____.

　A. Right　　　　　　B. Wrong　　　　　　C. Doesn't say

2. The nurse has to deal with the patient's postoperative nausea, which is very serious. _____.

    A. Right   B. Wrong   C. Doesn't say

3. Everyone feels the same about the postoperative pain. _____.

    A. Right   B. Wrong   C. Doesn't say

4. Playing games after an operation can ease the pain. _____.

    A. Right   B. Wrong   C. Doesn't say

5. If the patient has a sore throat, he needs to drink some hot water. _____.

    A. Right   B. Wrong   C. Doesn't say

Ⅱ Discussion.

What symptoms may the patient have after surgical operation?

Part 2 Short Passage

Urinary Catheterization

Urinary catheterization is the introduction of a catheter through the urethra into the bladder for the purpose of withdrawing urine. A catheter is a tube for injection or removing fluids. Catheterization is considered the most prominent cause of infection acquired in hospital. Whenever possible, it is recommended that catheterization should be avoided. When deemed necessary, it should be performed with careful techniques.

The following are common reasons for performing a urinary catheterization.

1. To relieve urinary retention.

2. To obtain a sterile urine specimen from a woman.

3. To measure the amount of post-void residual (PVR) urine in the bladder.

4. To obtain a urine specimen when a specimen cannot be secured satisfactorily by other means.

5. To empty the bladder before, during, and after surgery and before certain diagnostic examination.

Routine procedures of catheterizing the female bladder are as follows.

1. Assemble equipment. Wash hands, and explain the procedure and its purpose to the client. Protect the privacy by closing the curtain or door.

2. Assist the client to be in the dorsal recumbent position with the knees flexed and the feet about 2 feet apart.

3. Clean the perineal area with soap and warm water. Rinse and dry the area. Wash hands again.

4. Ask the client to lift her buttocks and slide the sterile drape under her. To avoid contamination, a sterile drape may be placed over the perineal area to expose the labia.

5. Open the supplies: a. If the catheter is to be indwelling, test the catheter balloon by prefilling with sterile water; b. Pour the antiseptic solution over cotton balls; c. Lubricate the catheter tip 1 to 2

inches deep in order to make the insertion more easier.

6. Spread the labia and identify the meatus. Clean both labia folds and the meatus. from front to back with cotton balls that are held with forceps. Move the cotton from above the meatus down toward her rectum. Place the end of the catheter in the receptacle.

7. Insert the catheter tip into the meatus 5 to 7.5 cm (2-3 inches) or until urine flows. For an indwelling catheter, once urine drains, advance the catheter another 2.5 to 5.0 cm.

8. Inject sterile water to inflate the balloon, hold the catheter securely.

9. Remove the equipment and record the time of the catheterization, the amount of urine removed, a description of the urine, and the client's reaction to the procedure.

🎧 Key Words

catheter / ˈkæθɪtə(r) / n. 导管
urethra / jʊˈriːθrə / n. 尿道
dorsal / ˈdɔːsl/ adj. 背部的
perineal / perɪˈniːəl / n. 会阴的
drape / dreɪp / n.（手术室的）消毒被单（或盖布）

labia / ˈleɪbiə / n. 阴唇
meatus / miˈeɪtəs / n. 道，口
forceps / ˈfɔːseps/ n. 手术钳
drainage / ˈdreɪnɪdʒ / n. 排水
receptacle / rɪˈseptəkl / n. 容器

Useful Expressions

urinary catheterization　导尿管插入术
post-void residual (PVR) urine　残尿

antiseptic solution　抗菌溶液
indwelling catheter　留置导管

Exercise

I Choose the best answer to each question based on the text.

1. Which one is Not the reason for catheterization?

  A. To empty the bladder before surgery

  B. To get a urine sample

  C. To avoid contamination

2. Dorsal recumbent position means _____.

  A. bending one's knees and lying on his/her back

  B. lying on one's side

  C. the prone position

3. From the context, we may figure out that the word "prominent" in the first paragraph means _____.

  A. severe   B. common   C. major

4. The purpose of lubricating the catheter tip is to _____.

  A. decrease the possibility of producing organism

  B. facilitate the insertion of the catheter

C. minimize the risk of contaminating the catheter

5. The sterile drape should be placed over the perineal area in order to _____.

   A. protect against contamination

   B. see the perineal area clearly

   C. protect bed linen from being wet

Ⅱ Read the passage again and put the following extracts in the correct order.

☐ **A** Lubricate the catheter tip 1 to 2 inches deep.

☐ **B** Clean and dry the perineal area.

☐ **C** Place the drainage end of the catheter in the receptacle.

☐ **D** Clean both of the labia folds and meatus with cotton balls and move from the meatus down toward the rectum.

☐ **E** Spread the labia and identify the meatus.

☐ **F** A sterile drape may be placed over the perineal area, exposing the labia.

☐ **G** Insert the catheter tip into the meatus 5 to 7.5 cm.

Part 3 Text

🎧 Postoperative Nursing

The postoperative period begins with the end of the surgery and the admission to a postanaesthesia care unit (PACU), also called the recovery room. Some patients who have received a local anaesthetic or undergone operative procedures and not required anaesthesia may be discharged from the operating room to their ward or home. The length of the postoperative period varies with the time required to recover from the stress and disruption caused by the surgery and anaesthesia. This period may last only a few hours, or it may extend for several months.

The postoperative period can be divided into two phases. The first phase is the immediate postoperative period and is characterized by the initial recovery from the stress of anaesthesia and surgery during the first postoperative hours. The second phase is the period of resolution and healing. This period may extend for months after the major surgery. In fact, there is no distinct dividing line between the initial phase of the postoperative recovery and the second phase with the understanding that the two periods overlap.

Take an acute appendicitis as an example.

Appendicitis is an inflammation of the appendix. No one is absolutely certain what the function of the appendix is. One thing we do know: we can live without it, without the appendix, we can still live with no apparent bad consequence. About 8% of the people in western countries have appendicitis at some time during their life, with a peak incidence between 10 and 30 years of age. The lumen Obstruction is believed to be the major cause of the acute appendicitis.

The classic symptoms of appendicitis include: (1) Dull pain near the navel of the upper abdomen becomes sharp as it moves to the lower right abdomen. (2) Nausea soon follows abdominal pain. (3) There is a swelling in the abdomen. (4) Fever ensues (low-grade fever), followed by the development of leukocytosis. (5) Coughing can cause increased pain.

In general, there are two treatment ways, including surgical treatment and non-surgical treatment. Most patients with acute appendicitis are managed by prompt surgical removal of the appendix except that the objective condition is not allowed—the serious organic disease. The postoperative nursing of appendicitis is as follows.

1. After surgery, the patient with lumbar hemp anaesthesia should lay down for 6-12 hours, no cushion pillow, to prevent the occurrence of postoperative headache. Observe vital signs. Measure blood pressure and pulse every hour.

2. If there is a drainage tube, change the patient's position into half-lying to facilitate the drainage and prevent the flow of inflammatory exudates into the abdominal cavity.

3. The patient was asked to fast and take the liquid on the day of the operation and gradually have soft diet on the second day after the operation. Under normal conditions, the patient can eat ordinary food on the third day.

4. After 24 hours, the patient can get out of bed to promote bowel movement, blood circulation and wound healing.

🎧 Key Words

disruption / dɪsˈrʌpʃn / n. 破坏；分裂
overlap / ˌəʊvəˈlæp / v. 部分重叠
appendicitis / əˌpendɪˈsaɪtɪs / n. 阑尾炎
lumen / ˈluːmen / n（管状器官内的）内腔
swelling / ˈswelɪŋ / n. 肿胀

ensue / ɪnˈsjuː/ vi. 跟着发生
leukocytosis / ˌluːkəʊsaɪˈtəʊsɪs / n. 白细胞增多
lumbar / ˈlʌmbə(r) / adj. 腰部的
hemp / hemp / n. 大麻制成的麻醉药

Useful Expressions

local anaesthetic　局部麻醉剂
be characterized by　以……为特点

lumbar hemp　腰麻

Exercise

Ⅰ Choose the best answer to each question based on the text.

1. How many symptoms of appendicitis does the text mention? _____.

　　A. 5　　　　　　　　　　B. 4　　　　　　　　　　C. 3

2. Who is NOT suitable for appendicitis surgery? _____.

　　A. The patient under the age of 3

　　B. A woman who is pregnant

　　C. The patient with severe heart disease

3. Appendix is an organ that is _____.

   A. very important   B. indispensable   C. not essential

4. "Fast" in the sentence "The patient was asked to fast... on the day of the operation" means to _____.

   A. walk fast   B. eat nothing   C. operate fast

5. The major cause of acute appendicitis is _____.

   A. cell aging   B. the development of leukocytosis

   C. blocking in the inner cavity

II Match each medical term in Column A with its explanation in Column B.

Column A	Column B
_____ 1. appendicitis	a. a gross increase in the number of white blood cells in the blood, usually as a response to an infection
_____ 2. leukocytosis	b. an illness in which a person's appendix is infected and painful
_____ 3. exudate	c. a substance that oozes out from animals or plants
_____ 4. recovery	d. gradual healing after sickness
_____ 5. obstruction	e. the state or condition of being blocked

III Find words or terms in the article to match the following definitions.

1. the feeling that you have when you want to vomit _____

2. a cavity or passage in a tubular organ _____

3. abnormal protuberance or localized enlargement _____

4. a small bag of tissue that is attached to the large intestine, which has no real function in humans

_____

IV Critical thinking.

According to the case at the beginning of this unit, what are nursing diagnoses and nursing interventions for the patient?

1. Nursing diagnoses

   • Pain related to the surgical procedure

   • Ineffective airway clearance related to anaesthesia or surgery

   • Altered nutrition: less than body requirement related to pain and loss of appetite

2. Nursing interventions

The nurse needs to explain to the patient about the postoperative pain and know about the pain relief ordered. The feeling of dizziness is a normal reaction to anaesthetic. The sore throat and thirstiness is caused by the nasogastric tube. Some ice chips can help relieve the discomfort. The patient requires the routine postoperative care including the frequent assessment of the respiration and the cardiovascular system and the assessment of the operation site.

Part 4 Supplementary Reading

🎧 Pain Scales

A pain scale measures a patient's pain intensity or other features. It's a universal pain assessment tool. This pain assessment tool is intended to help patient-care providers assess pain according to individual needs. Pain scales are available for neonates, infants, children, adolescents, adults, seniors and persons whose communication is impaired. There are several pain scales being used today ranging from numerical ones to graphics.

Numeric rating scale (NRC) is an 11-point scale for patient's self-reporting of pain. It is for adults and children of 10 years old or older.

0   No pain: feeling perfectly normal.

1   Mild: barely noticeable pain. Most of time, the pain can be ignored.

2   Discomforting: minor pain, like lightly pinching the fold of skin by using the fingernails.

3   Tolerable: very noticeable pain, like an accident cut. The pain is not so strong that one cannot get used to it.

4   Distressing: strong, deep pain like an average toothache. So strong that one notices the pain all the time and cannot completely adapt to it .

5   Very distressing: strong, deep, piercing pain such as a sprained ankle. Not only does one notice the pain all the time, but also his lifestyle is curtailed.

6   Intense: strong, deep pain. So strong that it seems to partially dominate one's sense, causing him to think somewhat unclearly.

7   Very intense: The pain completely dominates one's sense, causing him to think unclearly about half the time.

8   Utterly horrible: Pain is so intense that one can no longer think clearly at all. Suicide is frequently contemplated and sometimes tried.

9   Excruciating: Pain is so intense that one cannot tolerate it and demand pain killers or surgery.

10   Unimaginable: The consciousness can be lost as a result of the pain, such as a crushed hand in a severe accident.

Younger patients are asked to use wong-baker facial grimace scale chart to express pain intensity. Any patient from the age of around three can use the chart. It's also useful for patients who can't express themselves well enough in English to explain their pain level. Face 0 is very happy because he doesn't hurt at all. Face 1 hurts a little bit. Face 2 hurts a little more. Face 3 hurts even more. Face 4 hurts a whole lot. Face 5 hurts as much as one can imagine. Ask the patient to choose the face that best describes how he is feeling.

Exercise

Choose the best answer to each question based on the text.

1. Which of the following is true according to the passage? _____.

    A. Pain level 1-3 (mild pain)

    B. Pain level 4-6 (severe pain)

    C. Pain level 7-10 (moderate pain)

2. The word "impaired" in Paragraph 1 means _____.

    A. smoothed   B. damaged   C. blocked

3. If the patient is two years old, he should be asked to use _____ to express how painful he is.

    A. numeric rating scale

    B. wong-baker facial grimace scale chart

    C. both A and B

4. A pain scale tells us the patient's pain _____.

    A. site   B. intensity   C. tolerance

5. A 5-year-old child pointed to the third face to explain his pain. The nurse would understand that his pain was _____.

    A. mild pain   B. moderate pain   C. severe pain

Part 5 Medical Word Elements

1. oste(o)-	骨
osteoporosis /ˌɒstiəʊpəˈrəʊsɪs /	骨质疏松
osteoarthritis /ˌɒstiəʊɑːˈθraɪtɪs /	骨关节炎
2. vertebr(o)-	脊椎（柱）
vertebrectomy /ˌvɜːtɪˈbrekəmi /	椎骨切除术
vertebroarterial /ˌvɜːtɪbrəʊɑːˈtɪəriəl /	椎动脉的
3. angi(o)-	管的
angiocardiogram /ˌændʒɪəʊˈkɑːdiəgræm /	心血管造影片
angioedema /ˌændʒɪəʊiːˈdiːmə /	血管（神经）性水肿
4. gli(o)-	胶质
gliocyte /ˈglaɪəʊsaɪt /	神经胶质细胞
glioma /glaɪˈəʊmə /	神经胶质瘤
5. myel(o)-	脊髓
myelography /ˌmaɪəˈlɒgrəfi /	脊髓（X 线）造影术
myeloneuritis /ˌmaɪələʊnjʊəˈraɪtɪs /	脊髓神经炎
6. narc(o)-	麻醉，睡眠
narcolepsy /ˈnɑːkəlepsi /	发作性睡眠

narcotic / nɑːˈkɒtɪk /	麻醉的，麻醉药
7. spin(o)-	脊柱（椎）
spinogram / ˈspaɪnəgræm /	脊柱造影照片
spinothalamic / ˌspɪnəʊθəˈlaɪmɪk /	脊髓丘脑的
8. -ectomy	切除术
uterectomy / ˌjutəˈrektəmi /	子宫切除术
tylectomy / ˈtaɪlektəmi /	肿瘤切除术
9. -tomy	切开术
peritoneotomy / ˌperɪˌtəʊniˈɒtəmi /	腹膜切开术
hysterotomy / ˌhɪstəˈrɒtəmi /	子宫切开术

（陈 爽 赵 静）

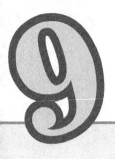

Caring for a Patient with Diabetes

Learning Objectives:

1. *Discussing diabetic management with patients*
2. *Describing the use of insulin pen*
3. *Defining and classifying the different types of diabetes mellitus*
4. *Explaining the importance of self-management in diabetes care*

Lead-In

Case Study

John Kim was a 52-year-old teacher who had non-insulin-dependent diabetes mellitus for 6 years. He was 67 inches (1.7 m) tall and weighed 202 pounds (91.6 kg). John had many misconceptions about diabetes, especially nutrition, stemming from experiences with his mother's diabetes. He usually skipped breakfast, had lunch and supper, and ate snacks in the evening, crackers, chips, and beer. To lose some weight, he went to the gym every day and tried some high intensity exercise. Recently, he always had a feeling of dizziness and anxiety; he also complained about tingling and numbness around the mouth; and he also had blurred vision and sweaty palm.

Part 1 Dialogue

🎧 Diabetes Education

Beth, the ward nurse, is talking to Mr. Kim about some diabetic management.

Beth: Hello, Mr. Kim. Nice to see you again.

Mr. Kim: Hello, Beth.

Beth: I'd like to talk to you today about the lifestyle and nutrition. You will have to make some major lifestyle changes if you're going to avoid complications of diabetes.

Mr. Kim: All right. I know I haven't been looking after my health lately. I've put on a bit of weight.

Beth: Mm, how many meals a day do you eat?

Mr. Kim: It depends. Sometimes I skip meals. I just can't be bothered.

Beth: Yeah, I know it must be difficult for you, but it's important that you eat small regular meals. You need to reduce your intake of saturated fats. Try to make sure you include carbohydrates in each meal.

Mr. Kim: Oh, I know. My daughter is always on about that, too.

Beth: You really should keep a close eye on your weight. How often do you exercise?

Mr. Kim: Not enough these days. I used to walk in the park after supper.

Beth: Could you try to include some physical activity in your daily routine? It would be a good idea to walk again.

Mr. Kim: Yes, I suppose so. All right, I'll make an effort to do that. Any other changes?

Beth: Yes, what's your alcohol intake like? How many drinks do you have per week?

Mr. Kim: I used to have a couple of beers in the evening, but I have been having a few more these days.

Beth: Well, look, alcohol in moderation isn't normally a problem. It can be a problem for diabetics, though. You must keep a close eye on your alcohol intake because it can affect your insulin dose.

Mr. Kim: Oh, all right. I'll keep an eye on it, as you say.

Beth: OK. Last question, it's an important one. How many cigarettes are you smoking at the moment?

Mr. Kim: A couple of packs a week. I know, I know. I'm trying to give up.

Beth: Good for you. It is hard but it is important to stop smoking if you want to avoid circulation problems.

Mr. Kim: I certainly don't want anything like that.

Beth: It's quite hard to quit on your own. You might like to speak to your doctor about some nicotine patches.

Mr. Kim: Thanks, I'll keep that in mind.

🎧 Key Words

diabetic / ˌdaɪə'betɪk / n. / adj. 糖尿病患者；糖尿病的

intake / 'ɪnteɪk / n. 吸收，摄入

carbohydrate / ˌkɑːbəʊ'haɪdreɪt / n. 碳水化合物

alcohol / 'ælkəhɒl / n. 酒精

insulin / 'ɪnsjʊlɪn / n. 胰岛素

dose / dəʊs / n. 剂量

circulation / ˌsɜːkjʊ'leɪʃn / n. 循环

Useful Expressions

saturated fat   饱和脂肪

keep a close eye on   密切注意……

physical activity   体力活动

nicotine patches   尼古丁戒烟贴片

Exercise

I **Read the dialogue again and decide whether the following statements are right or wrong. If there is not enough information to answer "Right" or "Wrong", choose "Doesn't say".**

1. The nurse is talking with Mr. Kim about diabetic management. _____.

    A. Right   B. Wrong   C. Doesn't say

2. Mr. Kim has a good control of his condition. _____.

    A. Right   B. Wrong   C. Doesn't say

3. Mr. Kim always walks in the park in order to lose weight. _____.

    A. Right   B. Wrong   C. Doesn't say

4. Alcohol intake can raise the blood glucose level. _____.

    A. Right   B. Wrong   C. Doesn't say

5. Mr. Kim must give up smoking to avoid lung problems. _____.

    A. Right   B. Wrong   C. Doesn't say

II **Discussion.**

What significant changes should Mr. Kim make to his lifestyle?

Part 2 Short Passage

Insulin Pen

An insulin pen is used to inject insulin for the treatment of diabetes. It is composed of an insulin cartridge and a dial to measure the dose, and is used with disposable pen needles to deliver the dose.

Insulin pens are used by 95% of insulin-treated patients in Europe, Asia, and Australia with excellent results. Insulin pens have a number of advantages.

1. More convenient and easier to transport than a traditional vial and syringe.

2. An insulin cartridge can fit into the device and can be changed.

3. Easier to use for those with visual or fine motor skill impairments.

4. Less injection pain (as polished and coated needles are not dulled by insertion into a vial of insulin before a second insertion into the skin).

Unlike the traditional syringe, two kinds of insulin cannot be mixed by the user in an insulin pen. In addition, using pens and pen needles is usually more expensive than using the syringe.

It is important that proper injection sites on the body be used. A health care provider helps determine the best injection site for a patient. In general, recommended injection sites include the abdomen, parts of the buttocks, parts of the upper arms and thigh areas.

To use the insulin pen properly, one should follow the procedure.

1. Before we start, we will wash our hands and get everything ready on the trolley. Then take the cover off the insulin pen.

2. Use an alcohol wipe to clean the rubber seal at the end of the insulin pen. After that, screw the needle at the end of the insulin pen.

3. Prime the pen to get the insulin right to the end of the needle. Turn the end of the pen to the number two.

4. Get the insulin to the end of the needle to prime the pen. Turn the end of the pen to dial the dose of insulin.

5. Pinch up some skin on your abdomen. Hold the pen up and inject into the raised skin. Hold the button at the end of the pen and count to five so that all the insulin can go in.

6. Remove used pen needle for disposal. Put the pen away for use next time.

🎧 Key Words

cartridge / ˈkɑːtrɪdʒ / n. 笔芯

disposable / dɪˈspəʊzəbl / adj. 一次性的

vial / ˈvaɪəl / n.（装药物等的）小瓶

syringe / sɪˈrɪndʒ / n. 注射器

visual / ˈvɪʒuəl / adj. 视力的

impairment / ɪmˈpeəmənt / n. 损伤

insertion / ɪnˈsɜːʃn / n. 插入

abdomen / ˈæbdəmən / n. 腹部

thigh / θaɪ / n. 大腿

prime / praɪm / vt. 装填

Useful Expressions

be composed of　由……构成

fine motor skills　精细动作运动技能

health care provider　医疗保健人员

Exercise

I **Choose the best answer to each question based on the text.**

1. An insulin pen is composed of a dial, a disposable needle and a(n) _____.

　　A. cartridge　　　　B. cover　　　　　　C. insulin

2. Which of the following is the advantage of insulin pen? _____.

　　A. Two types of insulin can be mixed

　　B. It is easy to carry

　　C. It is more expensive than the syringe

3. When choosing a proper injection site, _____ is recommended.

　　A. hand　　　　　　B. lower arm　　　　C. abdomen

4. After cleaning the rubber seal at the end of the insulin pen, one should _____.

　　A. prime the pen　　B. take the cover off　　C. screw the needle onto the end of the insulin pen

5. To make sure all the medicine has gone into the body, the best way is to _____.

　　A. press the injection site

B. hold the pen for several seconds

C. remove the needle as soon as possible

Ⅲ Read the passage again and put the following extracts in the correct order.

☐ **A** Pinch up skin and inject.

☐ **B** Take the cover off the insulin pen.

☐ **C** Clean the rubber seal of the insulin pen.

☐ **D** Screw the needle at the end of the insulin pen.

☐ **E** Hold the pen and count to 5.

☐ **F** Turn dose to 2 and prime the pen.

☐ **G** Turn the end of the pen to dial the dose.

Part 3 Text

🎧 Diabetes

Diabetes mellitus is a chronic and potentially disabling disease characterized by elevated blood sugar level. It causes alterations in the metabolism of carbohydrates, proteins, and fats. Generally, diabetes is due to dysfunction of pancreas which leads to insulin insufficiency. Insulin is necessary for body to use sugar. It is classified into two types: insulin-dependent diabetes and non-insulin dependent diabetes.

Insulin-dependent diabetes mellitus (IDDM) which is also called type I diabetes, develops during childhood or young adulthood. Type I diabetes may be slightly more prevalent in men than in women and tends to run in families. When diagnosed, individuals are often thin and have recently experienced excessive thirst (polydipsia), frequent urination (polyuria), feeling very hungry (polyphagia), and weight loss. Other common symptoms are: extreme fatigue; blurry vision; cuts/bruises that are slow to heal. Because individuals with IDDM produce no insulin, insulin therapy is essential to prevent rapid and severe dehydration, ketoacidosis, and death.

Non-insulin dependent diabetes mellitus (NIDDM) is also called type II diabetes. It can occur at any age but usually occurs after the age of 40. Most patients are obese or have a history of obesity at the time of diagnosis. Classic symptoms associated with diabetes are not present when first diagnosed. Although the symptomatology of type II diabetes is less obvious than that of type I, this classification is accompanied by vascular and neuropathic complications, such as tingling pain or numbness in the hands or feet. Typically, type II diabetics are not absolutely dependent on insulin for survival, although insulin therapy is often employed to lower blood glucose levels.

People living with diabetes may have to deal with short-term or long-term complications as a result of their condition. Short-term complications include hypoglycemia, diabetic ketoacidosis (DKA). Long-term complications include the eye problems (retinopathy), heart problems, nerves and feet problems. To decrease the risk of diabetes and the related complications, diabetes managements requires awareness. Make every meal well-balanced. Fruits, vegetables and whole grains are better than others. These foods are low in carbohydrates and contain fiber that helps keep blood sugar levels more stable. Choose nonfat dairy and lean meats. Limit foods that are high in sugar and fat. Sugar-sweetened beverages, such as soda, juice and sports drink, can be used as an effective treatment for quickly raising blood sugar that is too low. Physical activity is another important part of diabetes management plan. Regular exercise also helps the body use insulin more efficiently. Be aware of warning signs of low blood sugar, such as feeling shaky, weak, tired, hungry, lightheaded, and anxious. Always bring a small snack during exercise in case the blood sugar level drops too low. It's important to make major lifestyle changes to cope with the disease, such as giving up smoking, limiting the intake of alcohol, keeping a positive attitude, and remembering to have a regular check-up on eyes and feet.

🎧 Key Words

metabolism / mə'tæbə,lɪzəm / n. 新陈代谢

pancreas / 'pæŋkriəs / n. 胰腺

fatigue / fə'ti:g / n. 疲劳

bruise / bru:z / n. 挫伤；淤伤

dehydration / ,di:haɪ'dreɪʃn / n. 脱水

ketoacidosis / ,ki:təʊ,æsɪ'dəʊsɪs/ n. 酮症酸中毒

obesity / əʊ'bi:səti / n. 肥胖症

symptomatology / ,sɪmptəmə'tɒlədʒi / n. 症状；症状学

vascular / 'væskjələ(r) / adj. 血管的

neuropathic / ,njʊərə'pæθɪk / adj. 神经性的

hypoglycemia / ,haɪpəʊglaɪ'si:miə / n. 低血糖

retinopathy / retɪ'nɒpəθi / n. 视网膜病

Useful Expressions

diabetes mellitus　糖尿病

insulin-dependent diabetes mellitus (IDDM)　胰岛素依赖型糖尿病

non-insulin dependent diabetes mellitus (NIDDM)　非胰岛素依赖型糖尿病

run in families　家族遗传

food high/low in　高或低……的食物

give up smoking　戒烟

Exercise

▌ Choose the best answer to each question based on the text.

1. How many types of diabetes does the text mention? _____.

　A. 1　　　　　　　　　　B. 2　　　　　　　　　　C. 3

2. Which of the following is NOT the symptom of type I diabetes? _____.

　A. Eating more food　　B. Drinking more water　　C. Gaining more weight

3. A 16-year-old teenager who is 150 pounds (68.04 kg) in weight rarely does any exercise in his spare time. Which type of diabetes does he properly suffer from? _____.

　A. Type I diabetes　　　B. Type II diabetes　　　C. Both type I and type II diabetes

4. The following are effective ways to control diabetes except _____.

   A. keeping balanced diet

   B. taking regular exercise

   C. taking more insulin

5. A diabetic recently feels weak and tired. What should he do? _____.

   A. Give up smoking

   B. Eat some snacks during exercise

   C. Inject more insulin

II Match each medical term in Column A with its explanation in Column B.

	Column A	Column B
_____	1. polyuria	a. low blood sugar
_____	2. hypoglycemia	b. dryness due to the removal of water
_____	3. dehydration	c. increased urination
_____	4. obesity	d. an injury that results in some discolouration
_____	5. bruise	e. more than average fatness

III Find words or terms in the article to match the following definitions.

1. substances found in certain kinds of food that provide energy _____

2. a substance found in food and drink such as meat, eggs and milk _____

3. a large exocrine gland located behind the stomach _____

4. a disease of the retina that can result in the loss of vision _____

IV Critical thinking.

According to the case at the beginning of this unit, what are nursing diagnoses and nursing interventions for John Kim?

1. Nursing diagnoses

   • Knowledge deficit related to diabetes self-management

   • Risk for injury related to hypoglycemia attack

   • Risk for activity intolerance related to glycometabolism disorder

2. Nursing interventions

Patients' education is critical to the maintenance of normal blood glucose levels and the prevention of severe hypoglycemia episodes. Carefully assess and teach the patient about diabetes management. In addition, assist the patient in planning for the prevention of hypoglycemia episodes such as balanced food intake; careful monitoring and timing of meals and snacks; regular, sustained exercise; self-monitoring of blood glucose (SMBG) before and after exercise.

Part 4 Supplementary Reading

🎧 Hemodialysis

Hemodialysis is the mechanical process of removing waste products of protein metabolism, maintaining fluid and electrolyte balance, and restoring acid-base balance in patients with compromised renal function. Thus the hemodialysis machine becomes an artificial kidney, which may be used in the acute phase of renal failure, or to maintain life in the patient with chronic renal failure (CRF).

In simple terms, hemodialysis involves removing "unfiltered" blood from the patient; filtering out electrolytes, urea, creatinine, and so on through the dialysis process; and returning the "filtered" blood back to the patient. To remove and return the blood, vascular access is required, such as the cannulation of femoral or subclavian and the insertion of two single-lumen catheters or one large double-lumen catheter, surgical creation of an internal arteriovenous fistula or graft, or surgical creation of an external arteriovenous shunt. Besides vascular access, hemodialysis requires anticoagulation of the blood while it is outside the body and being filtered in the dialyzer. Hemodialysis may also incorporate the use of a mechanical pump that generates artificial pressure gradients across which fluid is filtered. Hemodialysis is the most efficient form of dialysis because of the rapidity of the process.

Patients in acute renal failure (ARF) may require daily hemodialysis; Hemodialysis usually lasts 3 to 5 hours and is performed three times per week. The patients with CRF may choose to be treated at a hemodialysis center or may opt for home care. Because the shunt, fistula and graft are vascular access sites necessary for dialysis, care must be taken to prevent compromised blood flow to the area. The patient is instructed not to wear tight clothing and not to sleep with his or her head on an arm. Signs are posted at the head of the patient's bed to alert health care personnel against taking blood pressure or performing venipunctures on the involved extremity. The access site is inspected for evidence of infection, and strict aseptic technique is used. The nurse must palpate for a thrill or auscultate for a bruit at the access site and notify the physician if a change indicates the potential thrombus formation or the clotting of the access site.

Exercise

Choose the best answer to each question based on the text.

1. Hemodialysis is used to treat the following conditions except _____.

    A. uremia   B. kidney failure   C. heart failure

2. Which of the following statements is NOT true according to the passage?_____.

    A. Hemodialysis is the most efficient way to cure chronic kidney disease.

B. The mechanism of hemodialysis is to remove and return blood.

C. During the process, electrolyte, urea and creatinine need to be removed.

3. What vascular access can be used for hemodialysis according to the passage? _____.

A. Peritoneal access

B. Continuous hemofiltration

C. Internal arteriovenous fistula

4. What is the advantage of hemodialysis? _____.

A. No blood loss   B. Rapid process   C. Continuous removal of fluid

5. Nursing instructions include that _____.

A. the patient should wear some tight clothes when undergoing dialysis

B. the nurse should take blood pressure on the involved extremity

C. the aseptic technique should be used to perform the procedure

Part 5 Medical Word Elements

1. immun(o)-	免疫
immunodeficiency / ˌɪmjuːnəʊdɪˈfɪʃənsi /	免疫缺陷
immunotherapy / ˌɪmjuːnəʊˈθerəpi /	免疫疗法
2. lymph(o)-	淋巴
lymphocyte / ˈlɪmfəsaɪt /	淋巴细胞
lymphoma / lɪmˈfəʊmə /	淋巴瘤
3. necr(o)-	坏死
necrosis / neˈkrəʊsɪs /	坏死
necrotic / neˈkrɒtɪk /	坏死的
4. thyr(o)-	甲状腺
thyroidism / ˈθaɪrɔɪdɪzəm /	甲状腺功能亢进
thyroiditis / ˌθaɪrɔɪˈdaɪtɪs /	甲状腺炎
5. poly-	多，多数
polyuria / ˌpɒlɪˈjuəriə /	多尿
polyphagia / ˌpɒlɪˈfeɪdʒiə /	多食症
6. -cyte	细胞
immunocyte / ˈɪmjuːnəʊsaɪt /	免疫细胞
monocyte / ˈmɒnəsaɪt /	单核细胞
7. gluc(o)-	葡萄糖
glucopenia / ˌgluːkəʊˈpiːniə /	低血糖
glucosuria / ˌgluːkəʊˈsjuəriə /	糖尿
8. glyc(o)-	糖，葡萄糖
glycoregulation / ˌglaɪkəʊˌregjuˈleɪʃn /	糖代谢调节

glycogenosis / ˌglaɪkədʒɪˈnəʊsɪs /　　　　　糖原贮积病，糖原病

9. nephr(o)-　　　　　　　　　　　　　　　　肾

　　nephremia / neˈfriːmiə /　　　　　　　　肾充血

　　nephrolithiasis / ˌnefrəʊlɪˈθaɪəsɪs /　　　肾结石

（赵　静）

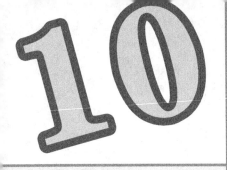

Caring for a Patient with Heart Disease

Learning Objectives:

1. *Discussing heart disease with patients*
2. *Describing electrocardiograph monitoring*
3. *Defining and classifying the different types of heart failure*
4. *Explaining the importance of cardiopulmonary resuscitation*

Lead-In

Case Study

Daniel Baza was a 64-year-old gentleman who had been treated for myocardial infarction and hypertension during the past 5 years. Today he presented himself in hospital with shortness of breath, which had been progressive over the past 3 days. He had experienced episodes of shortness of breath, especially when exerting himself. He also fatigued easily and complained of anorexia. Last night, he awoke from sleep because of sudden severe chest pain. His breathing was laboured and his lips had a blue tinge.

Part 1 Dialogue

🎧 Educating a Patient About Heart Disease

Mr. Baza is admitted to the hospital because of a recent heart attack. Christine, a ward nurse, is educating him about causes and precautions against heart disease.

Christine: How are you feeling today, Mr. Baza?

Mr. Baza: Hi, Christine. Much better. The chest pain seems to have disappeared.

Christine: I'm happy to hear that. Have you ever had this sort of pain before?

Mr. Baza: Never hurt like that. Well, five years ago in a routine check-up the doctor told me that I had myocardial infarction. But it didn't bother me and I could carry on as usual. About the last two years, I have noticed when I climb stairs my heart beats faster and I have to stop and catch my breath.

Christine: Don't worry. It is recommended that you temporarily not do exercise.

Mr. Baza: OK, I will. Could you tell me something more about heart disease?

Christine: Sure. Heart and blood vessel disease, called heart disease, includes many different forms.

The most common cause of heart disease is narrowing or blockage of the coronary arteries, the blood vessels that supply blood to the heart itself. This is called coronary artery disease. As time goes on, less and less oxygen enters the heart. It's the major reason why people have heart attacks.

Mr. Baza: What makes the coronary arteries become narrow?

Christine: It's plaque which builds up in the walls of the arteries. This buildup narrows the arteries, making it harder for blood to flow through. If a blood clot forms, it can stop the blood flow. This can cause a heart attack or a stroke.

Mr. Baza: I'm always short of breath when I go upstairs. Why does this happen?

Christine: A lack of oxygen would cause the person to become fatigue and easily tired.

Mr. Baza: No wonder I feel tired all the time.

Christine: There are many risk factors for heart disease, such as high blood pressure, high cholesterol, smoking, obesity and physical inactivity.

Mr. Baza: Maybe I should consider quitting smoking.

Christine: Smoking may double the risk of developing heart disease.

Mr. Baza: What else should I pay attention to?

Christine: The doctor ordered that you should stay in bed for several days, and if you feel any shortness of breath, please let me know. Your diet should be low in cholesterol and sodium. You should avoid defecation straining. I'll give you glycerin suppository to help you, or if necessary, I'll do the enema for you.

Mr. Baza: OK, I see. Thanks for the explanations.

Christine: You're welcome.

🎧 Key Words

myocardial / ˌmaɪəʊˈkɑːdiəl / adj 心肌的
infarction / ɪnˈfɑːkʃn / n. 梗死
cholesterol / kəˈlestərɒl / n. 胆固醇
blockage / ˈblɒkɪdʒ / n. 堵塞

coronary / ˈkɒrənri / adj. 冠状的，冠状动脉的
artery / ˈɑːtəri / n. 动脉
plaque / plæk / n. 血小板

Useful Expressions

heart attack　心脏病发作
routine check-up　常规体检

short of breath　呼吸短促
blood clot　血凝块，血块

Exercise

I **Read the dialogue again and decide whether the following statements are right or wrong. If there is not enough information to answer "Right" or "Wrong", choose "Doesn't say".**

1. The nurse is talking with Mr. Baza about heart disease. _____.

    A. Right   B. Wrong   C. Doesn't say

2. All was right in Mr. Baza's last routine check-up five years ago. _____.

    A. Right   B. Wrong   C. Doesn't say

3. Mr. Baza is always short of breath when he goes upstairs. _____.

    A. Right   B. Wrong   C. Doesn't say

4. A lack of oxygen would not cause the person to be tired. _____.

    A. Right   B. Wrong   C. Doesn't say

5. Mr. Baza didn't follow the doctor's order. _____.

    A. Right   B. Wrong   C. Doesn't say

II **Discussion.**

What should Mr. Baza do to avoid episodes of shortness of breath and chest pain?

Part 2 Short Passage

🎧 Electrocardiograph Monitoring

Electrocardiograph (ECG) monitoring refers to the continuous monitoring of the change of patient's vital signs, such as respiration, body temperature, blood pressure, oxygen saturation and pulse so as to take timely measures to improve the efficiency and reliability of treatment.

As it is of great significance in cardiovascular diagnose and treatment, nurses should master the procedures and be familiar with the emergency treatment measures.

Prepare items. What should be fully prepared inchldes electrocardiograph, electrocardiogram and plug connecting wire, electrode plate, 75% ethyl alcohol cotton ball, and blood pressure cuff.

1. Wash hands and wear a surgical mask.

2. Check the patient's name and connect the equipment.

3. Patient should be in a semi-Fowler's or horizontal position comfortably.

4. Wipe chest skin where electrode pads should be pasted with 75% ethyl alcohol cotton ball.

5. Paste the electrode pads and connect them to the correct position of the patient; choose the right cuff, and tie the cuff around the upper arm, at roughly the same vertical height as the heart.

6. Set the alarm limit and the measuring time.

7. Clean fingernails and finger skin, fix the fiber to the finger with a fixed set or clip and connect the wire to monitor the oxygen saturation.

8. Observe the number of breaths on the monitor screen and the patient's respiratory rate.

9. Tell the patient it's the end of the monitoring and turn off the equipment. Remove the pads and cuff, then wipe the skin with dry gauze.

10. Assist the patient in dressing.

11. Wash hands and keep records.

To set properly, the standard of the alarm value during the use of ECG monitoring principles should be followed. Focus on the changes of the patient's condition in order to make a discovery of the range of a life-threatening emergency. According to the actual situation of patients, set up the scientific and timely alarm adjustment to meet the needs of observation and treatment of the illness due to the doctor's advice.

There are also other requirements and warnings. Patients are advised not to move or get rid of electrode on their own. Cell phones are forbidden to use during the ECG monitoring process for preventing the interference of electric waves. The skin condition should be under guidance to avoid pain and itching.

🎧 Key Words

electrocardiograph / ɪˌlektrəʊˈkɑːdiəʊɡrɑːf / *n.*
心电图仪

monitoring / ˈmɒnɪtərɪŋ / *n.* 监控；检验，检查

ethyl / ˈeθɪl / *n.* 乙酸乙酯

pulse / pʌls / *n.* 脉搏

respiration / ˌrespəˈreɪʃn / *n.* 呼吸；呼吸作用

cardiovascular / ˌkɑːdɪəʊˈvæskjələ(r) / *adj.*
心血管的

emergency / iˈmɜːdʒənsi / *adj.* 紧急情况下使用的

alarm / əˈlɑːm / *n.* 警报；警报器

life-threatening / ˈlaɪfθretnɪŋ / *adj.* 威胁生命的

Useful Expressions

connecting wire   连接线

blood pressure cuff   血压计套袖

oxygen saturation   氧饱和度

Exercise

I **Choose the best answer to each question based on the text.**

1. Electrocardiograph monitoring refers to the continuous monitoring of _____.

   A. the change of a patient's mental condition

   B. the change of a patient's vital signs

   C. the change of a patient's physical exercise

2. Which of the following is the advantage of the electrocardiograph monitoring? _____.

   A. To set the standard of the alarm value

   B. To enable nurses to keep records

   C. To take timely measures to improve the efficiency and reliability of treatment

3. When a patient is having the electrocardiograph monitoring, _____ is recommended.

    A. horizontal position   B. vertical position   C. prone position

4. Focus on the changes of the patient's condition in order to _____.

    A. set the alarm limit

    B. master the procedures

    C. make a discovery of the range of a life-threatening emergency

5. Why are cell phones forbidden during the ECG monitoring process? _____.

    A. In order to focus on the changes of the patient's condition

    B. For preventing the interference of electric waves

    C. In order to set up the scientific and timely adjustment of the alarm

Ⅲ Read the passage again and put the following extracts in the correct order.

    ☐ **A** Observe the number of breaths and the patient's respiratory rate.

    ☐ **B** Connect the equipment.

    ☐ **C** Fix the fiber to the finger.

    ☐ **D** Wash hands and wear a surgical mask.

    ☐ **E** Paste the electrode pads and tie the cuff around the upper arm.

    ☐ **F** Set the alarm limit and the measuring time.

    ☐ **G** Wipe the chest skin with 75% ethyl alcohol cotton ball.

Part 3 Text

🎧 Heart Failure

Heart failure is a condition in which the heart can't pump enough blood to meet the body's needs. At present the prevalence of heart failure is a rising trend in China. According to statistics, among those over the age of 70, there is one in every ten people suffering from heart failure. Without early diagnosis and treatment, it will be quite harmful and even life-threatening to patients' health.

The patient's symptoms, medical history, and a complete physical exam can be used as diagnostic criteria for heart failure. Blood tests, electrocardiography, and chest radiography could be useful to determine the underlying cause. The most common symptoms of heart failure are shortness of breath when taking exercise even when lying down, fatigue and tiredness, swelling in legs, feet, ankles and abdomen, tachycardia and arrhythmia.

Heart failure is caused by many conditions that will damage the heart muscle, including coronary artery disease, heart attack, cardiomyopathy, and high blood pressure. According to the side of the heart involved, heart failure can usually be divided into left-sided heart failure, right-sided heart failure and congestive heart failure. In most cases, it affects the left side, the heart's main pumping chamber, the left ventricle first.

Though heart failure is potentially fatal, many treatments and methods are available to manage its symptoms, which can help patients live longer and enjoy more active lives. With stable mild symptoms, treatment generally consists of changing the lifestyle such as choosing the heart-healthy eating which limits sodium, saturated and trans fats, added sugars, and alcohol, taking part in moderate physical activities, and quitting smoking.

Medications are also effective in treating heart failure, including: aldosterone antagonist, angiotensin converting enzyme (ACE) inhibitors, angiotensin II receptor blockers (RBS), angiotensin receptor-neprilysin inhibitors (ARNIs), beta-blockers, blood vessel dilators, digoxin and diuretics.

If conditions get worse, surgery is an important step to fight heart failure. Bypass surgery can reroute blood around the blocked arteries to help patient's heart get the blood needed. Heart valve surgery can repair or replace the valves. Ventricular assist device can be used in the heart's left ventricle or right ventricle to help it pump blood to the rest of the body. Cardiac resynchronization therapy (CRT) will offer a pacemaker inserted in the heart which is used to maintain an adequate heart rate. If conditions are severe, heart transplant should be considered.

Caring for a patient with heart failure, a nurse should do nursing diagnoses and interventions on drug uses, safety and exercises, diet and nutrition, and psychological nursing. Firstly, when caring for a patient who has difficulties in breathing, the nurse should change the patient's body position if necessary. Continuous low flow oxygen should also be needed. Secondly, efficacy and adverse reactions of prescribed drugs should be controlled. Thirdly, comfort and encourage the patients to establish the confidence of conquering the disease. Stable mood can reduce the excitability sympathetic nerve. Finally, educate patients with a healthy diet and lifestyles.

🎧 Key Words

radiography / ˌrediˈɒgrəfi / n. X 光线照相术

arrhythmia / əˈrɪθmiə / n. 心律不齐，心律失常

cardiomyopathy / ˌkɑːdiəʊmaɪˈɒpəθi / n.
（尤指原发性的）心肌病

ventricle / ˈventrɪkl / n. 心室

inhibitor / ɪnˈhɪbɪtə(r) / n. 抑制剂

receptor / rɪˈseptə(r) / n. 受体

angiotensin / ˌændʒiəʊˈtensən / n. 血管紧张素

dilator / daɪˈleɪtə / n. 扩张药物

digoxin / daɪˈgɒksɪn / n. 地高辛

diuretic / ˌdaɪjuˈretɪk / n. 利尿剂

valve / vælv / n. 瓣膜

pacemaker / ˈpeɪsmeɪkə(r) / n. 起搏器

Useful Expressions

congestive heart failure　充血性心力衰竭

aldosterone antagonist　醛固酮拮抗剂

angiotensin converting enzyme (ACE)　血管
紧张素转换酶

beta-blocker　β- 受体阻滞剂

bypass surgery　心脏搭桥手术

cardiac resynchronization therapy (CRT)　心脏
再同步治疗术

sympathetic nerve　交感神经

Exercise

Ⅰ Choose the best answer to each question based on the text.

1. How many types of heart failure does the text mention? _____.

    A. 1   B. 2   C. 3

2. Which of the following is NOT the symptom of heart failure? _____.

    A. Shortness of breath

    B. Fatigue and tiredness

    C. Weight loss

3. Which of the following statements is NOT true according to the passage? _____.

    A. The prevalence of heart failure is a rising trend in China these years

    B. Heart failure can't be diagnosed on a complete physical exam

    C. Patients should be comforted and encouraged to establish the confidence of conquering heart failure

4. The following are effective ways to control heart failure except _____.

    A. enough rest   B. medications   C. surgery

5. Caring for a patient with heart failure, a nurse should NOT _____.

    A. make patients do exercise as much as possible

    B. change the patient's body position if necessary

    C. recommend a healthy diet and lifestyle

Ⅱ Match each medical term in Column A with its explanation in Column B.

	Column A	Column B
_____	1. tachycardia	a. to move an organ, piece of skin, etc., from one person's body and put it into another's as a form of medical treatment
_____	2. arrhythmia	b. a manner of living that reflects the person's values and attitudes
_____	3. transplant	c. an abnormal rate of muscle contractions in the heart
_____	4. lifestyle	d. a disorder (usually from unknown origin) of the heart muscle (myocardium)
_____	5. cardiomyopathy	e. abnormally rapid heartbeat (over 100 beats per minute)

Ⅲ Find words or terms in the article to match the following definitions.

1. a condition in which the heart can't pump enough blood to meet the body's needs _____

2. the heart's main pumping chamber _____

3. a surgery that can reroute blood around the blocked arteries to help the patient's heart get the blood needed _____

4. an electronic device inserted in the heart which is used to maintain an adequate heart rate _____

IV Critical thinking.

According to the case at the beginning of this unit, what are the nursing diagnoses and nursing interventions for the patient?

1. Nursing diagnoses
   - Risk for the impaired gas exchange related to the decreased cardiac output
   - Risk for the activity intolerance related to fatigue, and shortness of breath
   - Pain related to myocardial ischemia
2. Nursing interventions

The patient is immediately placed on bed with a cardiac monitor. The patient also needs oxygen inhalation through nasal catheter or oxygen mask. The nurse should maintain accurate intake and output records. Dietary sodium is restricted as ordered. The patient is placed in a high position to decrease venous reflux. It may be helpful to sit the patient upright, place a pillow at the patient's back.

Part 4 Supplementary Reading

🎧 Cardiopulmonary Resuscitation (CPR)

Cardiopulmonary resuscitation (CPR) is a lifesaving skill which can, through proper training, save one's life in many emergencies, including a heart attack or near drowning. The lack of oxygenated blood will cause brain damage in only a few minutes after heart and breathing stop. CPR can keep oxygenated blood flowing to the brain and other vital organs until more definitive medical treatment can restore a normal heart rhythm.

Before beginning CPR, determine if the individual is conscious. Shout and/or tap the shoulders of individual. If there is no response, call emergency response to see if someone is available to help. Meanwhile, call the local emergency number and then institute CPR within 3 minutes.

Compressions, airway, breathing (C-A-B) are steps of CPR.

Compressions: Restore blood circulation

1. Place the victim on firm surface, such as floor or ground.

2. Place the heel of one hand on the victim's breastbone, 2 finger-widths above the meeting area of the lower ribs, exactly between the normal position of the nipples. Place your second hand on top of the first hand, palms-down, interlock the fingers of the second hand between the first.

3. Compress chest downward hard to proper depth and then release at a rate of 80 to 100 compressions a minute. Use upper body weight while pushing straight down on the chest at least 5 centimeters but not greater than 6 centimeters. Do not take the heels of hands off the chest when releasing.

Airway: Open the airway

Make sure a foreign body that may obstruct the airway should be removed. Put a palm on the patient's forehead and tilt the head back gently. Then, gently lift the chin forward with the other hand to open the airway.

Breathing: Breathe for the person

1. Pinch the victim's nose with the thumb and the index finger and occlude the victim's mouth with the rescuer's mouth to perform mouth-to-mouth artificial respirations.

2. Give 2 rescue breaths after 30 chest compressions. Administer 1-second breaths mouth-to-mouth.

3. Lean over the victim's head and look at his/her chest to determine if the chest rise and fall. If not, resume another CPR cycle.

CPR can be terminated under the following conditions.

1. The resuscitation was successful.

2. Vital functions return spontaneously.

3. Assisted life-support measures are initiated.

4. Emergency medical personnel take over.

5. The rescuer is exhausted and could not continue.

Exercise

Choose the best answer to each question based on the text.

1. Cardiopulmonary resuscitation (CPR) can save one's life in many emergencies, including _____.

   A. heart attack   B. dehydration   C. hypoglycemia

2. Which of the following statements is true according to the passage? _____.

   A. Only emergency medical personnel can institute CPR

   B. Make sure a foreign body that may obstruct the airway should be removed

   C. During compressions the heels of the hands can be taken off chest when releasing

3. Before beginning CPR, what is the first thing to determine? _____.

   A. If the individual is conscious

   B. If the local emergency number has been called

   C. If there is someone available to help

4. What are the correct steps of CPR? _____.

   A. Compressions, calling, breathing

   B. Compressions, airway, breathing

   C. Compressions, calling, observing

5. CPR can be terminated under the following conditions, except that _____.

   A. the resuscitation was successful

   B. vital functions return spontaneously

   C. the rescuer thinks it's useless to continue

Part 5 Medical Word Elements

1. cardi(o)-   心脏的
   cardiogram / ˈkɑːdiəgræm /   心动图
   cardiopulmonary / ˌkɑːdiəʊˈpʌlmənəri /   心肺的
2. atri(o)-   心房
   atrioventricular / ˌeɪtrɪəʊvenˈtrɪkjulə /   房室的
   atriomegaly / ˈɑːtriəmegəli /   心房扩大
3. ventricul(o)-   室
   ventriculography / venˌtrɪkjuˈlɒgrəfi /   心/脑室造影术
   ventriculotomy / venˌtrɪkjuˈlɒtəmi /   心/室切开术
4. arteri(o)-   动脉
   arteriovenous / ɑːˌtiəriəʊˈviːnəs /   动静脉的
   arteriosclerosis / ɑːˌtɪəriəʊskləˈrəʊsɪs /   动脉硬化
5. ven(o)-   静脉
   venography / vɪˈnɒgrəfi /   静脉造影术
   venostasis / viːˈnɒstəsɪs /   静脉淤滞
6. vas(o)-   血管，管
   vasculopathy / ˌvæskjuˈlɒpəθi /   血管病
   vasopressor / ˌvæsəʊˈpresə /   血管加压药
7. sphygm(o)-   脉搏
   sphygmograph / ˈsfɪgməgrɑːf /   脉搏描记器
   sphygmometer / sfɪgˈmɒmɪtə /   脉搏计
8. intra-   在…内
   intracellular / ˌɪntrəˈseljuːlə /   细胞内的
   intravenous / ˌɪntrəˈviːnəs /   静脉注射的
9. hom(o)-   相同
   homosexual / ˌhəʊməˈsekʃuəl /   同性恋的；同性恋者
   homologous / həˈmɒləgəs /   同源的
10. heter(o)-   异
    heterogeneity / ˌhetərədʒəˈniːəti /   异质性
    heterotrophic / ˌhetərəˈtrəʊfɪk /   异养的

（刘　杨　赵　静）

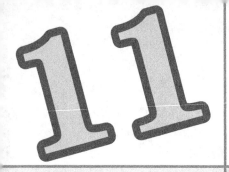

Caring for a Patient with Hepatitis

Learning Objectives:

1. *Discussing the transmitted routes, symptoms and treatment of hepatitis B with patients*
2. *Describing the procedures of blood transfusion*
3. *Basically introducing the viral hepatitis*
4. *Briefly explaining the symptoms and complications of AIDS*

Lead-In

Case Study

The patient was a previously healthy 44-year-old Mexican-American woman whose chief complaint was jaundice and right upper quadrant pain. For about 1 year, she had the sensation of a dry mouth. Over the next few weeks, she developed fatigue and a poor appetite. The following week she developed jaundice, right upper quadrant abdominal pain, dark urine, and clay-coloured stool. At this point in time, the patient saw a physician and was told that she had hepatitis. She was given esomeprazole, promethazine, clotrimazole, and rofecoxib.

Part 1　Dialogue

🎧 Educating a Patient About Hepatitis

Betty, a charge nurse on the Hepatology Department, is talking to Susan, a 44-year-old patient, about her hepatitis B. She has been admitted after her first serious hepatitis B attack and needs education about managing her condition.

Susan:　I'm here to fetch my physical examination report.

Betty:　Yeah, here it is.

Susan:　Could you explain it to me?

Betty:　Certainly. The blood test shows that you had leukocytosis, and increased alanine aminotransferase (ALT) and aspartate aminotransferase (AST). Hepatitis B surface antigen test is positive.

Susan:　What does it mean?

Betty: It means that you have hepatitis B.

Susan: I knew little about it. What should I do next?

Betty: Now I'm going to tell you something about hepatitis B. You can also ask some questions about it.

Susan: OK.

Betty: Hepatitis is caused by one of the five viruses that have been designated hepatitis A, B, C, D and E. The symptoms are similar for all the forms of viral hepatitis but the routes of infection are different. Hepatitis B is spread by blood or body fluids from an infected person. A baby can get it from its mother during childbirth, and it can also be spread by sexual contact, using street drugs, and unsafe medical care.

Susan: Any other transmitted routes?

Betty: Hepatitis B can also be caused or worsened by non-viral substances such as alcohol, medications and chemicals.

Susan: I even don't know how I've got it. Can you tell me its symptoms?

Betty: The person with hepatitis B will have the following symptoms: fatigue, mild fever, abdominal pain, muscle or joint pain, dark urine, pruritus, nausea, vomiting and loss of appetite. Some patients develop jaundice, in which the skin and the whites of the eyes appear yellow.

Susan: It seems that I've had almost all the symptoms.

Betty: However, hepatomegaly, cirrhosis, and hepatoma may eventually develop. These complications result in the death of 15% to 25% of those with this chronic disease.

Susan: Betty, I'm eager to know how to treat hepatitis B.

Betty: Some antiviral medications are helpful to patients with persistently elevated ALT levels by route of parenteral infusions when in a acute stage. As for diet, patients should eat foods with high protein, high carbohydrates and low fat in frequent small meals.

Susan: Can hepatitis B be prevented?

Betty: Hepatitis B can be prevented by vaccine, but there is no cure for it. You may relieve the symptoms by having a good rest, eating more nutritious foods, avoiding alcohol and cigarettes, and reducing stress from work.

Betty: Well, I understand. Thanks a lot.

🎧 Key Words

alanine / ˈælənin / n. 丙氨酸

aminotransferase / əˌmiːnəʊˈtrænsfəreɪs / n. 转氨酶

aspartate / əˈspaːteɪt / n. 天冬氨酸盐

antigen / ˈæntɪdʒən / n. 抗原

designate / ˈdezɪgneɪt / vt. 把······定名为

pruritus / prʊˈraɪtəs / n. 瘙痒

jaundice / ˈdʒɔːndɪs / n. 黄疸

hepatomegaly / hepətəʊˈmegəli / n. 肝肿大

cirrhosis / səˈrəʊsɪs / n. 肝硬化

hepatoma / ˌhepəˈtəʊmə / n. 肝细胞瘤

Useful Expressions

alanine aminotransferase (ALT)　丙氨酸氨基转移酶	surface antigen　表面抗原
aspartate aminotransferase (AST)　天门冬氨酸氨基	body fluid　体液
转移酶	dark urine　小便黄赤

Exercise

I　Read the dialogue again and decide whether the following statements are right or wrong. If there is not enough information to answer "Right" or "Wrong", choose "Doesn't say".

1. If your hepatitis B surface antigen test is positive, it means you have hepatitis B. _____.

　　A. Right　　　　　　　B. Wrong　　　　　　　C. Doesn't say

2. The symptoms of all forms of viral hepatitis are similar and the routes of infection are nearly the same. _____.

　　A. Right　　　　　　　B. Wrong　　　　　　　C. Doesn't say

3. Eventually, patients with hepatitis B will certainly develop hepatomegaly, cirrhosis or hepatoma. _____.

　　A. Right　　　　　　　B. Wrong　　　　　　　C. Doesn't say

4. Three complications of hepatitis B result in the death of 15% to 25% of those with this disease. _____.

　　A. Right　　　　　　　B. Wrong　　　　　　　C. Doesn't say

5. For patients with persistently elevated ALT levels, it's helpful to take some antiviral medications. _____.

　　A. Right　　　　　　　B. Wrong　　　　　　　C. Doesn't say

II　Discussion.

For a patient with hepatitis B, what should he/she pay special attention to in daily life?

Part 2　Short Passage

Blood Transfusion

Blood transfusion is generally the process of receiving blood or blood products into one's circulation intravenously. Transfusions are used for various medical conditions to replace lost components of the blood. Early transfusions used the whole blood, but the modern medical practice commonly uses only components of the blood, such as erythrocyte, leukocyte, plasma, clotting factors, and platelets.

Before a blood transfusion is given, there are many steps taken to ensure the quality of the blood products, compatibility, and safety to the recipient. The World Health Organization (WHO) recommends that all donated blood be tested for transfusion transmissible infections, including HIV, hepatitis B, hepatitis C, syphilis and other infections that pose a risk to the safety of the blood supply. All the donated blood should also be tested for the ABO blood group system and

RH blood group system to ensure that the patient is receiving compatible blood.

The following is how to administer a blood transfusion through a Y-set:

1. Close all the clamps on the Y-set.
2. Rotate the blood unit bag gently.
3. Pull back the tabs on the blood unit bag and expose the port.
4. Spike the port and carefully hang the unit.
5. Spike the small saline bag with other spike of the Y-tubing.
6. Hang the saline bag and the blood bag on the IV pole.
7. Open the clamp to the saline bag and squeeze the sides of the drip chamber until the filter is half covered and the drip chamber is full.
8. Open the main clamp and *prime* the rest of the tubing. Remove the cap that protects the end of the IV tubing.
9. *Replace* the cap and close the main clamp when the tubing is primed.
10. Cleanse the injection port on the primary IV.
11. Affix a large-gauge needle to the end of the tubing and the prime needle.
12. Insert the needle into the injection port and the clamp off the primary IV flow.
13. Open the clamp to the saline bag and turn the clamp on the main tubing.
14. Clamp off the saline bag and open the clamp to the blood bag.
15. Squeeze the sides of the Y-set drip chamber so that blood can cover the entire filter.
16. Administer the blood slowly for the first 15 minutes, approximately 20 drops per minute, or 100 mL/hr.
17. Observe the patient closely for reactions, chilling, backache, headache, nausea or vomiting, tachycardia, tachypnoea, skin rash, or hypotension.
18. Administer the blood unit at the prescribed rate if no adverse effects occur.
19. Complete the blood transfusion in less than 4 hours.
20. Monitor the patient throughout the transfusion.
21. Flush the lines with normal saline when the transfusion is completed.
22. Reattach the primary IV solution, and adjust the drip to the desired rate.
23. Remove the blood unit bag and the administration set.

🎧 Key Words

erythrocyte / ɪˈrɪθrəsaɪt / *n.* 红细胞
leukocyte / ˈljuːkəʊsaɪt / *n.* 白细胞
plasma / ˈplæzmə / *n.* 血浆
platelet / ˈpleɪtlət / *n.* 血小板

transmissible / trænzˈmɪsəbl / *adj.* 可传染的
syphilis / ˈsɪfɪlɪs / *n.* 梅毒
saline / ˈseɪlaɪn / *adj.* 含盐的

Useful Expressions

clotting factor   凝固因子
human immunodeficiency virus (HIV)   艾滋病病毒（人类免疫缺损病毒）
blood unit bag   血袋（常用规格为每袋 200 mL 或 400 mL）

skin rash   皮疹
drip chamber   滴注器；排水室，沉淀池

Exercise

I Choose the best answer to each question based on the text.

1. In modern medical practice, the most common way of blood transfusion is to _____.

    A. use whole blood

    B. use only components of the blood

    C. use only serum intravenously

2. According to the passage, which is NOT one of the steps taken to ensure the quality of the blood products, compatibility, and safety to the recipient? _____.

    A. Taking the temperature of the patient

    B. Testing for transmissible infections

    C. Testing for the ABO and RH blood group systems

3. The italicized word "prime" on page 103 probably means _____.

    A. being the first in rank or degree   B. to get something ready

    C. being at the best stage of development

4. The italicized word "replace" on page 103 probably means _____.

    A. to take the place of something

    B. to change something with a newer or better one

    C. to put something back

5. According to the passage, which of the following is NOT true? _____.

    A. The WHO recommends that all the donated blood be tested for syphilis

    B. In the process of the blood transfusion, the purpose of squeezing the sides of the Y-set drip chamber is to make blood cover the entire filter

    C. As long as the blood of the donator is compatible with the recipient, the blood transfusion can be administered

II Read the passage again and put the following extracts in the correct order.

☐ **A** Open the clamp to the saline bag and squeeze the sides of the drip chamber until the filter is half covered and the drip chamber is full.

☐ **B** Squeeze the sides of the Y-set drip chamber so that blood can cover the entire filter.

☐ **C** Reattach the primary IV solution, and adjust the drip to the desired rate.

☐ **D** Rotate the blood unit bag gently.

☐ **E** Affix a large-gauge needle to the end of the tubing and the prime needle.

☐ **F** Hang both the saline bag and the blood bag on the IV pole.

☐ **G** Observe the patient closely for reactions.

☐ **H** Administer the blood unit at the prescribed rate if no adverse effects occur.

Part 3 Text

🎧 Hepatitis

Any type of inflammation in the liver is called hepatitis. The most common cause of hepatitis worldwide is viruses. Other causes include heavy alcohol use, certain medications, toxins, other infections, autoimmune diseases, and non-alcoholic steatohepatitis (NASH). Hepatitis may be either acute or chronic.

There are five main types of viral hepatitis: Type A, B, C, D, and E. Hepatitis A is transmitted through fecal-oral route, usually by consuming food or beverage contaminated with fecal matter containing the virus. The concentration of Hepatitis A virus (HAV) in the stool of the infected person is the highest during the 2-week period before the onset of jaundice. Hepatitis B is transmitted through blood and body fluid. It is easy to catch and can be spread by sharing razors or needles by tattooing or body piercing, and from mother to infant during pregnancy or childbirth. Hepatitis C is spread in ways that are similar to hepatitis B. Hepatitis D can only infect people already infected with hepatitis B.

Hepatitis A, B, and D are preventable with immunization. Medications may be used to treat chronic cases of viral hepatitis. There is no specific treatment for NASH; however, a healthy lifestyle, including physical activity, a healthy diet, and weight loss, is important. Autoimmune hepatitis may be treated with medications to suppress the immune system. A liver transplant may also be an option in certain cases.

Hepatitis may present completely asymptomatic (12%-35% of the cases), with signs of chronic hepatopathy, or acute or even fulminant hypohepatia. People usually have one or more nonspecific symptoms, sometimes of long lasting duration, as fatigue, general ill health, lethargy, headache, weight loss, dull pain in right upper quadrant (RUQ), repugnance to food, malaise, anorexia, lymphadenectasis, hepatomegaly, nausea, jaundice or arthralgia affecting the small joints. Rarely, rash, pruritus or unexplained fever may appear.

People with hepatitis should avoid taking drugs metabolized by the liver. Glucocorticoids are not recommended as a treatment option for acute viral hepatitis and may even cause harm, such as the development of chronic hepatitis.

Universal precautions should be observed, but isolation is not strictly necessary; isolation may be needed in cases of fecal incontinence in hepatitis A and E and uncontrolled bleeding in hepatitis B and C.

People with hepatitis should be encouraged to pay attention to the followings.

1. Ingest diet and fluid appropriately to promote liver regeneration.
2. Maintain a proper rest and limited activity to reduce metabolic workload of liver.
3. Keep a good personal hygiene habit to prevent contamination.
4. Avoid: alcohol, blood donation, and any OTC medication, esp. acetaminophen and sedatives for 3-12 months, sexual activity until antibody testing results are negative.
5. A follow-up case referral may take 6 months for recovery.
6. Instruct the contacts about available immunization.

🎧 Key Words

steatohepatitis / ˌstɪətəʊˌhepəˈtaɪtɪs / n. 脂肪肝

hepatopathy / ˌhepəˈtɒpəθi / n. 肝病

fulminant / ˈfʊlmɪnənt / adj. 暴发的

hypohepatia / ˌhaipəʊhɪˈpætiə / adj. 肝功能不全；
肝功能减退

nonspecific / ˌnɒnspəˈsɪfɪk / adj. 非特异性的

lethargy / ˈleθədʒi / n. 嗜睡

repugnance / rɪˈpʌɡnəns / n. 厌恶

anorexia / ˌænəˈreksiə / n. 神经性厌食症

lymphadenectasis / lɪmˌfædɪˈnektəsɪs / n. 淋巴结肿大

arthralgia / ɑːˈθrældʒiə / n. 关节痛

glucocorticoid / ˌɡluːkəʊˈkɔːtɪkɔɪd / n. 糖皮质激素

acetaminophen / əˌsiːtəˈmɪnəfen / n. 对乙酰氨基酚

Useful Expressions

body piercing   人体穿孔艺术

dull pain   隐痛

right upper quadrant (RUQ)   右上腹

fecal incontinence   大便失禁

liver regeneration   肝再生

Exercise

Ⅰ Choose the best answer to each question based on the text.

1. Hepatitis D can only infect people already infected with _____.

    A. hepatitis A   B. hepatitis B   C. hepatitis C

2. Hepatitis C may be spread in one of the following ways except _____.

    A. through blood and body fluid

    B. through sharing razors or needles by tattooing or body piercing

    C. through kissing

3. What kind of hepatitis is transmitted through fecal-oral route? _____.

    A. Hepatitis A   B. Hepatitis B   C. Hepatitis C

4. According to the text, which of the following is NOT true? _____.

    A. Hepatitis A, B, and D are preventable with immunization

    B. Isolation of hepatitis patients is completely unnecessary

    C. It's of importance for the patients with hepatitis to have a good rest and limited activity to reduce metabolic workload of liver

5. For the patient with NASH, it is important for him/her to _____.

    A. find a specific medicine   B. take acetaminophen

    C. have a healthy lifestyle

Ⅱ Match each medical term in Column A with its explanation in Column B.

	Column A	Column B
_____	1. toxin	a. a piece of solid waste from your bowels
_____	2. stool	b. not showing any symptoms of the disease
_____	3. transmitted	c. one of four equal parts
_____	4. quadrant	d. a poisonous substance
_____	5. asymptomatic	e. infected

III **Find words or terms in the article to match the following definitions.**

1. a general feeling that you are slightly ill or not happy in your life _____

2. a drug used to make someone calm or go to sleep _____

3. the proportion of essential ingredients or substances _____

4. being in a medical condition in which normal cells are attacked by the body's immune system _____

5. a state of not having much energy or enthusiasm _____

IV **Critical thinking.**

According to the case at the beginning of this unit, what are the nursing diagnoses and the nursing interventions for the patient?

1. Nursing diagnoses

 • Fatigue related to increased energy demands

 • Risk for infection related to the disease process and transmission of hepatitis

 • Altered nutrition related to anorexia and difficulty of digesting fats

2. Nursing interventions

Nurses must take actions to prevent the spread of hepatitis. Conduct isolation precautions such as blood and body fluid precautions. It's important that the patient should get an adequate amount of rest. A high-carbohydrate, low-fat diet is more tolerated. The nurse observes and records the amount and the colour of urine and stool. Soap and rubbing alcohol are avoided because they will further dry the skin.

Part 4 Supplementary Reading

🎧 Acquired Immunodeficiency Syndrome

Acquired immunodeficiency syndrome (AIDS) results from the infection with a virus called human immunodeficiency virus (HIV). This virus infects key cells in the human body called CD4-positive (CD4+) T cells. These cells are part of the body's immune system, which fights infections and various cancers. HIV infection is mainly transmitted through sexuality, blood or from a mother to a baby.

AIDS symptoms of infection perform variously in the internal organs and in different parts of the tumour. In the following areas general symptoms include persistent fever, weakness, night sweats, general superficial lymphadenopathy, weight loss; respiratory symptoms: long-term cough, chest pain, dyspnoea, sputum serious blood; gastrointestinal symptoms: such as anorexia, nausea, vomiting, diarrhoea, severe blood in the stool; the nervous system symptoms: dizziness, headache, unresponsiveness, decreased intelligence, mental disorders, twitch, hemiplegia and dementia; damage to the skin and mucous membranes: diffuse papules, herpes zoster, inflammation and ulceration on oral and pharyngeal mucosa. Therefore, the symptom of AIDS is very complex.

Some AIDS's complications include: 1. Kaposi's sarcoma (KS) that represents red or purple maculae, papules. 2. CMV retinitis—a virus that infects the back of the eye. 3. Pneumocystis carinii pneumonia (PCP)—a type of pneumonia, an infectious disease of the lung. 4. Toxoplasmosis—a disease caused by a parasite, which can cause problems in the brain as well as other systems in the body. 5. Invasive cervical cancer—cancer of the bottom part of a woman's uterus.

The diagnosis of HIV infection can be made by detecting antibodies in the blood. Two different types of antibody tests, enzyme-linked immunoassay (ELISA) and Western blot, are available.

Medicines called antiretrovirals help people with AIDS. Other five most important HIV medicines are: stavudine, lamivudine, nevirapine, zidovudine and efavirenz.

HIV is NOT spread by:

- Body fluids like saliva (spit), tears, or sweat
- Touching a person with HIV (like shaking hands or hugging)
- Sharing dishes or drinking from the same glass used by someone with HIV
- Light switches or toilet seats
- Drinking fountains
- Air or water
- Insects, like mosquitoes

Psychologically, common misconceptions about AIDS and HIV are diminishing. However, the stigma of the condition persists in many parts of the world. People who are living with HIV may feel excluded, rejected, discriminated, and isolated.

There is currently no vaccine or cure for HIV or AIDS. People living with HIV should improve their general health by regularly exercising, eating healthfully, and not smoking. They should also be especially cautious to prevent exposure to infection.

Exercise

Choose the best answer to each question based on the text.

1. Which of the following is NOT right according to the text? _____.

   A. AIDS is an infectious disease   B. Our immune system includes CD4-positive T cells

   C. AIDS can be transmitted by touching a person with HIV

2. Of the AIDS symptoms, which of the following is right? _____.

   A. Respiratory symptoms include hemiplegia and dementia

   B. The nervous system symptoms include general superficial lymphadenopathy

   C. Damage to the skin and mucous membranes includes herpes zoster

3. Some AIDS's complications include _____.

   A. KS—a virus that infects the back of the eye

   B. CMV retinitis—a type of pneumonia, an infectious disease of the lung

   C. Toxoplasmosis —a disease which can cause problems in the brain

4. HIV can be spread _____.

   A. by sharing dishes or drinking from the same glass used by someone with HIV

   B. by insects, like mosquitoes

C. through blood

5. According to the passage, we know _____.

    A. though common misconceptions about AIDS and HIV are diminishing, the stigma of the condition persists in many parts of the world

    B. the passage introduces 3 different types of antibody tests and 5 most important HIV medicines

    C. women with AIDS are encouraged to have children

Part 5 Medical Word Elements

1. hepat(o)-	肝
hepatoma / ˌhepəˈtəʊmə /	肝脏肿瘤
hepatomegaly / ˌhepətəʊˈmegəli /	肝肿大
2. chole, chol(o)-	胆汁
cholecyst / ˈkɒləsɪst /	胆囊
chololith / ˈkɒləlɪθ /	胆石
3. pancreat(o)-	胰（腺）
pancreatography / ˌpænkriəˈtɒɡrəfi /	胰腺造影（术）
pancreatotropic / ˌpæŋkriətəʊˈtrɒpɪk /	促胰腺的
4. splen(o)-	脾
splenodynia / ˌspliːnəʊˈdɪniə /	脾痛
splenoptosis / ˌspliːnəʊˈtəʊsɪs /	脾下垂
5. abdomin(o)-	腹
abdominalgia / ˌæbdɒmɪˈnældʒiə /	腹痛
abdominoscopy / æbˌdɒmɪˈnɒskəpi /	腹腔镜检查
6. gastr(o)-	胃
gastratrophia / ˌɡæstrəˈtrəʊfiə /	萎缩性胃炎
gastrostomy / ɡæsˈtrɒstəmi /	胃造口术
7. -osis	病，病态
coniosis / ˌkəʊnɪˈəʊsɪs /	粉尘病
tuberculosis / tjuːˌbɜːkjuˈləʊsɪs /	肺结核
8. -pathy	疾病
thrombopathy / θrɒmˈbɒpəθi /	血小板（功能）紊乱
cardiomyopathy / ˌkɑːdiəʊmaɪˈɒpəθi /	心肌病
9. sub-	下
subcutaneous / ˌsʌbkjuˈteɪniəs /	皮下的
subarachnoid / ˌsʌbəˈræknɔɪd /	蛛网膜下腔的
10. super-	超
superego / ˌsjuːpəˈiɡəʊ /	超我
superinfection / ˌsjuːpərɪnˈfekʃn /	重复感染

（余 可 赵 静）

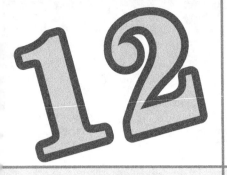

Caring for a Child with Pneumonia

Learning Objectives:

1. *Discussing the function and structure of the respiratory system with patients*
2. *Describing how to use a pediatric oxygen tent*
3. *Defining and classifying pneumonia*
4. *Understanding and explaining the ventilator*

Lead-In

Case Study

A 10-year-old girl developed fever, headache and malaise for 4 days followed by a nonproductive cough and scratchy throat. On examination, her temperature was 39.6 ℃, pulse 90 beats/min, blood pressure 110/70 mmHg, respiratory rate 20 beats/min. Physical examination was unremarkable except for scattered rales over the left lower lung, and small bullae in her left tympanic membrane. Chest X-ray revealed a patchy left lower lobe infiltrates. At the doctor's request, she made a heroic effort but was unable to produce sputum.

Part 1 Dialogue

🎧 Describing Respiratory System

Betty, a charge nurse on the Pediatric Respiratory Ward, is describing the function and structure of the respiratory system to 10-year-old Susan, who has been suffering from asthma.

Betty: Hi, Susan. You're feeling much better than yesterday, aren't you? We'll chat with you about your breathing now, and then I'll talk to you about what's happening to your airways when your asthma attacks. OK ?

Susan: OK!

Betty: Susan, I wish you can understand what happens to you during an asthma attack, so that you can deal with it when another asthma attacks.

Susan: Yeah, go on please.

Betty: Now, look at this little booklet's first page, and you'll see a diagram of the respiratory system. I'll tell you how the air comes into our bodies and travels to our lungs.

Susan: I'm eager to know it.

Betty: First, I will tell you the functions of the respiratory system and what the respiratory system is made up of. Then I will talk about what happens normally, and how the air will move into our lungs.

Susan: OK.

Betty: The function of the respiratory system is the intake of oxygen and the removal of carbon dioxide. It also helps regulate the balance of acid and base in tissues. Our airway is divided into the upper respiratory tract and the lower respiratory tract. The former consists of nose, pharynx, larynx and trachea and the latter includes bronchi, bronchioles and lungs. Can you see that?

Susan: Interesting!

Betty: The air is sucked into your nasal cavity where it's warmed and filtered. It moves past the oral cavity. Now it goes through your pharynx, and then comes to the epiglottis. The tube which carries food to your stomach is right next to it, so that part is like a road which divides into two roads.

Betty: Great! Now the air is moving past your larynx down into your trachea, or windpipe, and into the bronchi. That's the part which swells when you have an attack. We'll talk about what happens in an asthma attack later, OK?

Susan: OK. What happens to the air now?

Betty: Well, see how the bronchus is divided into the two lungs? The lungs are covered by pleural membrane. That's the special covering that protects your lungs. Inside the lungs are the alveoli, which are masses of tiny sacs which help your lungs to exchange carbon dioxide for oxygen. Then you can breathe out the carbon dioxide.

Susan: I get it now.

🎧 Key Words

asthma / ˈæsmə / n. 哮喘
diagram / ˈdaɪəgræm / n. 图表
regulate / ˈregjuleɪt / v. 调节
pharynx / ˈfærɪŋks / n. 咽
larynx / ˈlærɪŋks / n. 喉
trachea / trəˈkiːə / n. 气管
bronchi / ˈbrɒŋkaɪ / n. 支气管（bronchus 的复数）

bronchiole / ˈbrɒŋkɪəʊl / n. 细支气管
epiglottis / ˌepɪˈglɒtɪs / n. 会厌
windpipe / ˈwɪndpaɪp / n. 气管
pleural / ˈplʊərəl / adj. 胸膜的
alveoli / ælˈviːəlaɪ / n. 肺泡（alveolus 的复数）
sac / sæk / n. 囊，液囊

Useful Expressions

respiratory system　呼吸系统
intake of oxygen　氧气吸入
carbon dioxide　二氧化碳

balance of acid and base　酸碱平衡
upper respiratory tract　上呼吸道

Exercise

I　Read the dialogue again and decide whether the following statements are right or wrong. If there is not enough information to answer "Right" or "Wrong", choose "Doesn't say".

1. The function of the respiratory system is the intake of oxygen and the removal of carbon dioxide and it helps regulate the balance of acid and base in tissues. _____.

   A. Right　　　　　　B. Wrong　　　　　　C. Doesn't say

2. Our airway is divided into the left respiratory tract and the right respiratory tract. _____.

   A. Right　　　　　　B. Wrong　　　　　　C. Doesn't say

3. The upper respiratory tract consists of nose, pharynx, larynx and trachea. _____.

   A. Right　　　　　　B. Wrong　　　　　　C. Doesn't say

4. The air is sucked into your chest cavity where it's warmed and filtered. _____.

   A. Right　　　　　　B. Wrong　　　　　　C. Doesn't say

5. The common cold, also known as the upper respiratory tract infection, usually lasts about 5 to 7 days. _____.

   A. Right　　　　　　B. Wrong　　　　　　C. Doesn't say

II　Discussion.

How is the air inhaled into the lungs and exhaled out of the lungs normally?

Part 2　Short Passage

🎧 Using a Pediatric Oxygen Tent

Oxygen therapy, also known as supplemental oxygen, is the use of oxygen as a medical treatment. It can treat low blood oxygen, carbon monoxide toxicity, cluster headaches, the occurrence of chronic bronchitis or emphysema and maintain enough oxygen while inhaled anaesthetics are given. Long-term oxygen intake is often useful in people with chronically low oxygen such as from severe chronic obstructive pulmonary disease (COPD) or cystic fibrosis. Oxygen can be given in a number of ways including nasal cannula, face mask, oxygen tent and inside a hyperbaric chamber.

The following procedures will show how to use a pediatric oxygen tent.

1. Secure the tent and place the machine properly at the head of the bed.

2. Connect the regulator into the oxygen source.

3. Plug the machine in.

4. Set up the humidifier and make sure that the water level (the tray at the back of machine) is adequate.

5. Pad the frame that supports the canopy.

6. Turn on the oxygen to the desired concentration (30%-50%), and maintain the temperature

at 17.8-21.2 ℃ (64.0-70.0 ℉).

7. Secure the canopy by tucking in all sides and maintaining closure whenever possible.

8. Analyze and record the tent atmosphere, and check the child's vital signs every 12 hours.

9. Leave the crib sides up for safety.

10. Select toys that are washable without producing static electricity, and that are appropriate to the child's age.

11. Assist in placing on cardiac or apnoea monitor.

12. Keep the child warm and check the dampness of clothes.

13. Change bed linen and child's clothing whenever necessary.

Oxygen is required for normal cell metabolism. Excessively high concentrations can cause oxygen toxicity such as lung damage or result in respiratory failure in those who are predisposed. The target oxygen saturation which is recommended depends on the condition which the child is being treated in. In most conditions a saturation of 94%-98% is recommended, while in those at risk of carbon dioxide retention saturations of 88%-92% are preferred, and in those with carbon monoxide toxicity or cardiac arrest they should be as high as possible. Air is typically 21% oxygen by volume while oxygen therapy increases this by some amount up to 100%.

Oxygen is used as a medical treatment in both chronic and acute cases, and can be used in hospital, pre-hospital or post-hospital, dependent on the needs of the patient and their medical professionals' opinions. Oxygen is also widely used in emergency medicine.

🎧 Key Words

toxicity / tɒk'sɪsəti / n. 毒性
emphysema / ˌemfɪ'si:mə / n. 肺气肿
cystic / 'sɪstɪk / adj. 胆囊的；膀胱的
fibrosis / faɪ'brəʊsɪs / n. 纤维变性
cannula / 'kænjʊlə / n. 套管

hyperbaric / ˌhaɪpə'bærɪk / adj. 高气压的，高压的
pediatric / ˌpi:dɪ'ætrɪk / adj. 儿科的
canopy / 'kænəpi / n. 罩盖
apnoea / æp'ni:ə / n. 呼吸暂停；窒息
predispose / ˌpri:dɪ'spəʊz / adj. 易患……的

Useful Expressions

carbon monoxide   一氧化碳
oxygen saturation   氧饱和度

respiratory failure   呼吸衰竭
cardiac arrest   心脏停搏

Exercise

I Choose the best answer to each question based on the text.

1. Oxygen can be given in a number of ways including the following except _____.

　　A. nasal cannula and face mask 　　　　　　B. oxygen tent and inside a hyperbaric chamber

　　C. vein and artery

2. When using a pediatric oxygen tent, the desired oxygen concentration should be _____ and the temperature should be maintained at _____.

A. 30%-50%; 17.8-21.2 ℃   B. 50%-70 %; 21.8-26.2 ℃

C. 70%-90%; 26.8-31.2 ℃

3. The nurse giving oxygen therapy should check child's vital signs every _____.

A. 4 hours   B. 8 hours   C. 12 hours

4. If there is a risk of carbon dioxide retention, oxygen saturations of _____ are preferred.

A. 94%-98%   B. 88%-92%   C. 92%-96%

5. Oxygen is used as a medical treatment in _____.

A. both chronic and acute cases   B. both benign and malignant tumour treatment

C. both primary and secondary case

Ⅱ Read the passage again and put the following extracts in the correct order.

☐ **A** Turn on the oxygen to the desired concentration.

☐ **B** Assist in placing on cardiac or apnoea monitor.

☐ **C** Place machine properly at the head of the bed.

☐ **D** Set up the humidifier and check.

☐ **E** Leave the crib sides up for safety.

☐ **F** Plug the machine in.

☐ **G** Record the tent atmosphere, and check the child's vital signs.

☐ **H** Keep the child warm and dry.

Part 3 Text

🎧 Pneumonia

Childhood pneumonia is an inflammation or infection of the bronchioles and alveolar spaces of the lungs. It occurs most in infants and young children. It occurs most often in late winter and early spring. In China, pneumonia is still a leading cause of death among children.

Pneumonia can be classified according to morphology, etiology, and clinical forms. Clinically pneumonia may occur as either a primary disease or as a complication of some other illnesses, in which case it is termed secondary pneumonia. Morphologically pneumonia is recognized as lobar pneumonia, bronchopneumonia and interstitial pneumonia. In infants, pneumonia tends to remain bronchopneumonia with poor consolidation of alveoli. In older children, pneumonia may localize in a single lobe, and consolidation or infiltration of exudates into the alveoli may occur. Based on the etiologic agent, pneumonia can be classified into viral pneumonia, mycoplasma pneumonia, bacterial pneumonia and pneumonia associated with the aspiration of foreign substances.

The pneumococcus is the chief organism causing pneumonia in infants and early childhood. The onset of pneumococcal pneumonia is generally abrupt, following an upper respiratory tract infection. Symptoms and signs include fever, malaise, rapid and shallow respirations, cough, nasal flaring, retractions, chills, dyspnoea, and chest pain that is often exaggerated by deep breathing. The cough is dry at first, but gradually becomes productive. Fever rises as high as 103 ℉ to 104 ℉, and the child may have a febrile convulsion. Sternal retractions are brought into use which may be seen as the assisting muscles of respiration. Physical assessment will reveal tachypnoea and tachycardia because the lung space will be filled with exudates, and the respiratory function will be diminished. The breath sounds will become bronchial. Percussion will reveal dullness over a lobe where consolidation has occurred. Rales will be present. Laboratory studies will reveal leukocytosis. Chest X-ray will reveal patchy diffusion in young children and lung consolidation in older children.

Antibiotics and sulfonamides begin early in the disease. This is continued for 4 or 5 days after the temperature drops. Penicillin G is the drug usually ordered, because it is extremely effective against pneumococci. The infants may need an antipyretic such as aspirin or Tylenol to reduce fever. Oxygen is administered for dyspnoea or cyanosis. Intravenous therapy may be necessary to supply fluid, because the infant tires so readily with sucking that he cannot achieve a good oral intake.

The nursing diagnosis related to the child with pneumonia includes impaired gas exchange, ineffective airway clearance, ineffective breathing pattern, hyperthermia, risk for fluid volume deficit, and activity intolerance.

The nursing goals of the child with pneumonia are: to promote rest, maintain the patent airway, ease respiratory efforts, control fever, prevent dehydration, provide nutrition, monitor respiratory status, reduce anxiety and apprehension, and detect complications early.

Upon their child's discharge from the hospital, parents receive written instructions concerning diet, activity, medication, return appointments, and so on, and it is helpful if the parents repeat these instructions to the nurse so that the nurse may determine whether they have interpreted them correctly.

🎧 Key Words

morphology / mɔːˈfɒlədʒi / n. 形态学
etiology / ˌiːtiˈɒlədʒi / n. 病因学
lobar / ˈləʊbə / adj. 肺叶的
interstitial / ˌɪntəˈstɪʃl / adj. 间质的
consolidation / kənˌsɒlɪˈdeɪʃn / n. 巩固，凝固
infiltration / ˌɪnfɪlˈtreɪʃn / n. 渗透
mycoplasma / ˌmaɪkəʊˈplæzmə / n. 支原体

pneumococcus / ˌnjuːmə(ʊ)ˈkɒkəs / n. 肺炎球菌
（复数 pneumococci）
malaise / məˈleɪz / n. 不舒服
dyspnoea / dɪspˈniːə / n. 呼吸困难
antipyretic / ˌæntɪpaɪˈretɪk / n. 退热剂
cyanosis / ˌsaɪəˈnəʊsɪs / n. 发绀
hyperthermia / ˌhaɪpəˈθɜːmiə / n. 高热

Useful Expressions

secondary pneumonia　继发性肺炎
viral pneumonia　病毒性肺炎
bacterial pneumonia　细菌性肺炎

febrile convulsion　发热性惊厥
sternal retraction　胸骨凹陷
patchy diffusion　斑片状扩散

Exercise

I Choose the best answer to each question based on the text.

1. Based on the etiologic agent, pneumonias can be classified into several kinds. Which of the following is NOT one of them? _____.

    A. Viral pneumonia   B. Bacterial pneumonia   C. Secondary pneumonia

2. Which of the following is the chief factor causing pneumonia in infants and early childhood? _____.

    A. Pneumococcus   B. Bronchial inflammation

    C. Upper respiratory tract infection

3. Fever caused by pneumonia in infants and early childhood rises as high as _____.

    A. 100 ℉ to 102 ℉   B. 103 ℉ to 104 ℉   C. 106 ℉ to 107 ℉

4. Infants with pneumonia may need an antipyretic such as _____ to reduce fever.

    A. antibiotics and sulfonamides   B. penicillin G   C. aspirin or Tylenol

5. Oxygen is administered to the infants with pneumonia for _____ .

    A. dyspnoea or cyanosis   B. tachypnoea or tachycardia

    C. rapid and shallow respirations or chest pain

II Match each medical term in Column A with its explanation in Column B.

Column A	Column B
_____ 1. tachycardia	a. difficult or labored respiration
_____ 2. dyspnoea	b. abnormally high body temperature
_____ 3. hyperthermia	c. abnormally rapid heartbeat
_____ 4. leukocytosis	d. study of diseases' causes
_____ 5. etiology	e. abnormally increased white blood cells

III Find words or terms in the article to match the following definitions.

1. abnormally rapid respiration _____

2. any medicine that lowers the body temperature to prevent or alleviate fever _____

3. bacterium causing pneumonia in mice and humans _____

4. medical drugs used to kill bacteria and treat infections _____

IV Critical thinking.

    According to the case at the beginning of this unit, what are the nursing diagnoses and the nursing interventions for the patient?

1. Nursing diagnoses

    • Impaired gas exchange related to ventilation-perfusion mismatch or arteriovenous shunting

    • Alteration in the body temperature related to infection

    • Sleep pattern disturbance related to frequent coughing

2. Nursing interventions

Hypoxemia is an early sign of impaired gas exchange, and it must be identified and treated early to prevent the development of respiratory failure. Administration of oxygen may be appropriate for hypoxemia. The body temperature must be monitored closely and appropriate antibiotic therapy and antipyretic therapy must be implemented. The family members should guarantee the sufficient nutrients to meet the energy needs.

Part 4 Supplementary Reading

🎧 Ventilators

A medical ventilator is a mechanical ventilator, a machine designed to move breathable air into and out of the lungs, to provide breathing for a patient who is physically unable to breathe, or breathing insufficiently.

Ventilators are chiefly used in intensive care unit (ICU), home care, and emergency medicine and in anaesthesia (as a component of an anaesthesia machine).

In its simplest form, a modern positive pressure ventilator consists of a compressible air reservoir or turbine, air and oxygen supplies, a set of valves and tubes, and a disposable or reusable "patient circuit". The air reservoir is pneumatically compressed several times a minute to deliver room-air, or in most cases, an air/oxygen mixture to the patient. If a turbine is used, the turbine pushes air through the ventilator, with a flow valve adjusting pressure to meet patient-specific parameters. When overpressure is released, the patient will exhale passively due to the lungs' elasticity, the exhaled air being released usually through a one-way valve within the patient circuit called the patient manifold.

Ventilators may also be equipped with monitoring and alarm systems for patient-related parameters (e.g. pressure, volume and flow) and ventilator function (e.g. air leakage, power failure and mechanical failure), backup batteries, oxygen tanks, and remote control. The pneumatic system is nowadays often replaced by a computer-controlled turbopump.

Modern ventilators are electronically controlled by a small embedded system to allow exact adaptation of pressure and flow characteristics to an individual patient's needs. Fine-tuned ventilator settings also serve to make ventilation more tolerable and comfortable for the patient. In Canada and the United States, respiratory therapists are responsible for tuning these settings, while biomedical technologists are responsible for the maintenance.

The patient circuit usually consists of a set of three durable, yet lightweight plastic tubes, separated by function (e.g. inhaled air, patient pressure and exhaled air). Determined by the type of the ventilation needed, the patient-end of the circuit may be either non-invasive or invasive.

Non-invasive methods, which are adequate for patients who require a ventilator only while sleeping and resting, mainly employ a nasal mask. Invasive methods require intubation, which will normally be a tracheotomy cannula for long-term ventilator dependence, as this is much more comfortable and practical for long-term care than is larynx or nasal intubation.

Choose the best answer to each question based on the text.

1. Ventilators are NOT chiefly used in _____.

    A. intensive care unit (ICU) and emergency medicine

    B. home care and anaesthesia

    C. nursery school and nursing home

2. A medical ventilator is a machine designed to _____.

    A. move breathable air into and out of the lungs

    B. carry oxygen into and out of the brain

    C. carry blood into and out of the heart

3. Determined by the type of ventilation needed, the patient-end of the circuit may NOT be _____.

    A. non-invasive   B. invasive   C. semi-invasive

4. Non-invasive methods, which are adequate for patients who require a ventilator only while _____, mainly employ a nasal mask.

    A. sleeping and resting   B. sitting and standing

    C. lying and running

5. Invasive methods require intubation, which for _____ will normally be a tracheotomy cannula.

    A. short-term ventilator dependence   B. long-term ventilator dependence

    C. mid-term ventilator dependence

Part 5 Medical Word Elements

1. -pnea   呼吸
    apnea / æpˈniːə /   呼吸暂停
    eupnea / juːpˈniːə /   平静呼吸

2. pneum(o)-   肺
    pneumococci / ˌnjuːməˈkɒksaɪ /   肺炎球菌
    pneumonia / njuːˈməʊniə /   肺炎

3. trache(o)-   气管
    tracheostoma / treɪkiːˈɒstəmə /   气管造口
    tracheostomy / ˌtreɪkiˈɒstəmi /   气管切开术

4. nas(o)-   鼻
    nasogastric / ˌneɪzəʊˈgæstrɪk /   鼻胃的
    nasopharyngeal / ˌneɪzəʊfəˈrɪndʒiːəl /   鼻咽的

5. bronch(o)-   支气管
    bronchodilator / brɒŋkəʊdaɪˈleɪtə /   支气管扩张器
    bronchospasm / ˈbrɒŋkəˌspæzəm /   支气管痉挛

6. laryng(o)-   喉
    laryngoscope / ləˈrɪŋgəskəʊp /   喉头镜

laryngostenosis /lə,rɪŋəʊstɪ'nəʊsɪs/ 喉狭窄

7. pharyng(o)- 咽
   pharyngolaryngitis /fə,rɪŋəʊ,lærɪn'dʒaɪtɪs/ 咽喉炎
   pharyngodynia /fæ,rɪŋəʊ'dɪnɪə/ 咽痛

8. tachy- 快速
   tachycardia /,tækɪ'kɑːdɪə/ 心动过速，心搏过速
   tachypnea /,tækɪp'niːə/ 呼吸急促

9. brady- 徐缓
   bradyarthria /,brædɪ'ɑːθrɪə/ 言语迟缓，迟语症
   bradykinesia /,brædɪkɪ'niːzɪə/ 运动徐缓

10. dys- 困难
    dysfunction /dɪs'fʌŋkʃn/ 功能障碍
    dysphagia /dɪs'feɪdʒɪə/ 吞咽困难

（王炎峰　赵　静）

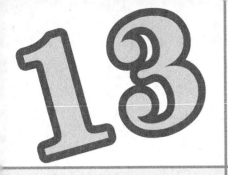

Caring for a Patient with Diarrhoea

Learning Objectives:

1. *Describing the process of digestion*
2. *Explaining intravenous therapy and the procedures of intravenous infusion*
3. *Defining and classifying different types of diarrhoea and its treatment*
4. *Defining and classifying different types of electrolyte and explaining its functions*

Lead-In

Case Study

A 10-month infant suffered from diarrhoea after he was fed some un-boiled bean curd two days ago. The stools were yellow waterish without any blood, defecation 10-15 times a day. No vomiting present. The physical examination showed the baby had got a high temperature of 38.5 ℃, Pulse 120 beats per minute. The baby also got dry lips, mild abdomen swelling, bowel sounds 10-12 times per minute, no high notes.

Part 1 Dialogue

🎧 Describing the Process of Digestion

Karen, a charge nurse on the Digestive Ward, is describing the normal digestion of food to Helen, a 9-year-old patient, who was admitted after having acute diarrhoea.

Karen : Hello, Helen. You are looking a bit brighter than yesterday. We'll have a chat about your digestion, as there are a few things you need to know.

Helen: OK. What do I have to know?

Karen : Look at this diagram that shows you the food digestion in your gastrointestinal tract, or GIT.

Helen: I understand, that includes mouth, stomach and intestines.

Karen : Yes. Digestion begins in the mouth with the secretion of saliva and its digestive enzymes.

Helen: When I am chewing the food, the mouth will produce saliva.

Karen: Right. Then, food is formed into a bolus and swallowed into the esophagus, from where it enters the stomach through the action of peristalsis.

Helen: Mm, peristalsis means the contraction of muscles.

Karen: That is right. Stomach secretes gastric juice which contains hydrochloric acid, pepsin and other digestive enzymes.

Helen: What do they do?

Karen: In the stomach further release of enzymes breaks down the food further and this is combined with the churning action of the stomach. The partially digested food enters the duodenum as a thick semi-liquid chyme.

Helen: Oh, chyme is thick semi-liquid.

Karen: Yes. Next, in the small intestine, the larger part of digestion takes place and this is helped by the secretions of bile, pancreatic juice and intestinal juice. The intestinal walls are lined with villi, and their epithelial cells are covered with numerous microvilli to improve the absorption of nutrients by increasing the surface area of the intestine.

Helen: Oh, I understand. What happens to the food next?

Karen: In the large intestine, the passage of food is slower to enable fermentation to take place by the gut flora. Here water is absorbed and waste material stored as feces to be removed by defecation via the anal canal and anus.

Helen: Why do I have diarrhoea?

Karen: The most common cause is an infection of the intestines due to virus, bacteria, or parasite——a condition also known as gastroenteritis.

Helen: What can cause infection?

Karen: These infections are often acquired from food or water that has been contaminated by feces, or directly from another person who is infected.

Helen: How can I prevent diarrhoea?

Karen: Diarrhoea can be prevented by improved sanitation, clean drinking water, and hand washing with soap.

Helen: Ok, I remember that.

🎧 Key Words

diarrhoea / ˌdaɪəˈrɪə / n. 腹泻，痢疾
digestion / daɪˈdʒestʃən / n. 消化
gastrointestinal / ˌɡæstrəʊɪnˈtestɪnl / adj. 胃肠的
secretion / sɪˈkriːʃn / n. 分泌
saliva / səˈlaɪvə / n. 唾液
bolus / ˈbəʊləs / n. 食团，小而圆的物块
esophagus / ɪˈsɒfəɡəs / n. 食管，食道
peristalsis / ˌperɪˈstælsɪs / n. 蠕动
hydrochloric / ˌhaɪdrəˈklɒrɪk / adj. 含氯化氢的，盐酸的

pepsin / ˈpepsɪn / n. 胃蛋白酶
churning / ˈtʃɜːnɪŋ / n. 搅拌
duodenum / ˌdjuːəˈdiːnəm / n. 十二指肠
semi-liquid / ˈsemiˈlɪkwɪd / adj. 半液体的；半流质的
chyme / kaɪm / n. 食糜
villi / ˈvɪlaɪ / n. 绒毛（villus 的复数）
epithelial / ˌepɪˈθiːlɪəl / adj. 上皮的；皮膜的
defecation / ˌdefəˈkeɪʃn / n. 排便
parasite / ˈpærəsaɪt / n. 寄生虫
gastroenteritis / ˌɡæstrəʊˌentəˈraɪtɪs / n. 肠胃炎

contaminated / kən'tæmɪneɪtɪd / *adj.* 受污染的；弄脏的　　　sanitation / ˌsænɪ'teɪʃn / *n.* 环境卫生；卫生设备

Useful Expressions

gastrointestinal tract (GIT)　消化道　　　　hydrochloric acid　盐酸
digestive enzyme　消化酶　　　　　　　　　anal canal　肛管
gastric juice　胃液

Exercise

I　Read the dialogue again and decide whether the following statements are right or wrong. If there is not enough information to answer "Right" or "Wrong", choose "Doesn't say".

1. Food bolus is swallowed into the esophagus and enters the stomach through the action of peristalsis. _____.

　　A. Right　　　　　　　B. Wrong　　　　　　　C. Doesn't say

2. Gastric juice secreted by stomach contains hydrochloric acid, pepsin and mucus. _____.

　　A. Right　　　　　　　B. Wrong　　　　　　　C. Doesn't say

3. The partially digested food enters the duodenum as a thick semi-liquid chyme. _____.

　　A. Right　　　　　　　B. Wrong　　　　　　　C. Doesn't say

4. Numerous microvilli covering on the epithelial cells improve the absorption of nutrients by decreasing the surface area of the intestine. _____.

　　A. Right　　　　　　　B. Wrong　　　　　　　C. Doesn't say

5. Diarrhoea can be prevented by improved sanitation, clean drinking water, and hand washing with soap. _____.

　　A. Right　　　　　　　B. Wrong　　　　　　　C. Doesn't say

II　Discussion.

What functions does each part of the digestive system have?

Part 2　Short Passage

🎧 Intravenous Therapy

　　Intravenous (IV) therapy is a therapy that delivers liquid substances directly into a vein. The intravenous route of administration can be used for injections (with a syringe at higher pressures) or infusions (typically using only the pressure supplied by gravity). Intravenous infusions are commonly referred to as drips. The intravenous route is the fastest way to deliver medications and fluid replacement throughout the body, because the circulation carries them. Intravenous therapy may be used for fluid replacement (such as correcting dehydration), to correct electrolyte imbalances, to deliver medications, and for blood transfusions.

A standard IV infusion set consists of a pre-filled, sterile container (glass bottle, plastic bottle or plastic bag) of fluids with an attachment that allows the fluid to flow one drop at a time, making it easy to see the flow rate (and also reducing air bubbles); a long sterile tube with a clamp to regulate or stop the flow; a connector to attach to an access device; and Y-sets to allow "piggybacking" of another infusion set onto the same line, e.g., adding a dose of antibiotics to a continuous fluid drip.

The procedures of IV infusion with pump are as follows.

1. Get the IV bag ready.

2. Before starting, wash hands.

3. Check the IV solution against the IV prescription.

4. Check the IV bag against the IV prescription.

5. To prime the line, run the IV fluid through the IV tubing of the giving set.

6. The giving set has one end to go into the IV bag and the other end is for connection to the patient's cannula.

7. Run the IV infusion through an IV infusion pump.

8. Set the rate on the infusion pump.

9. Start the infusion pump and pump is just for running a test.

10. Connect the IV to the patient's cannula.

11. Start the infusion.

12. Sign the IV prescription and write up the IV infusion on the Fluid Balance Chart.

IV therapy can cause complications such as infection, infiltration, fluid overload, electrolyte imbalance and so on. Infection symptoms are warmth, swelling, pain, and redness around IV sites or the vein (phlebitis). Infiltration is characterized by coolness and pallor to the skin as well as localized swelling or edema. Possible consequences of fluid overload include hypertension, heart failure, and pulmonary edema. Large amounts of cold fluids accidentally induced hypothermia, even ventricular fibrillation. A blood clot or other solid mass, as well as an air bubble, can be delivered into the circulation through an IV and end up blocking a vessel, called embolism.

🎧 Key Words

infusion / ɪnˈfjuːʒn / n. 输液
gravity / ˈɡrævəti / n. 重力
piggybacking / ˈpɪɡibækɪŋ / n. 搭载
prescription / prɪˈskrɪpʃn / n. 处方

phlebitis / fləˈbaɪtɪs / n. 静脉炎
edema / ɪˈdiːmə / n. 水肿
embolism / ˈembəlɪzəm / n. 栓塞

Useful Expressions

intravenous (IV) therapy　静脉治疗
intravenous infusion　静脉输液
fluid replacement　补液
electrolyte imbalance　电解质紊乱

blood transfusion　输血
fluid balance chart　体液平衡表
ventricular fibrillation　心室纤维性颤动

Exercise

I Choose the best answer to each question based on the text.

1. Which of the following descriptions about IV therapy is NOT true? _____.

   A. The intravenous route is the fastest way to deliver medications

   B. Intravenous infusions are commonly referred to as drips

   C. IV therapy delivers liquid substances directly into an artery

2. Intravenous therapy may NOT be used for _____.

   A. correcting dehydration   B. blood filtration

   C. correcting electrolyte imbalance

3. What does the word "piggybacking" in the second paragraph mean? _____.

   A. Riding on someone's shoulders or back   B. Resembling pig

   C. Providing approval and support

4. A standard IV infusion set consists of the following except _____.

   A. a long sterile tube   B. X-sets

   C. a pre-filled, sterile container

5. IV therapy can cause complications such as _____.

   A. infection, infiltration, fluid overload, electrolyte imbalance

   B. hypertension, heart failure, pulmonary edema

   C. hypothermia, even ventricular fibrillation

II Read the passage again and put the following extracts in the correct order.

   ☐ **A** Connect the IV to the patient's cannula.

   ☐ **B** Write up the IV infusion on the Fluid Balance Chart.

   ☐ **C** Sign the IV prescription.

   ☐ **D** Start the infusion.

   ☐ **E** Wash hands thoroughly.

   ☐ **F** Set the rate on the infusion pump.

   ☐ **G** Prime the line of the giving set.

   ☐ **H** Check the IV solution and the IV bag.

Part 3 Text

🎧 Diarrhoea

Diarrhoea, also spelled diarrhea, is the condition of having at least three loose or liquid bowel movements each day. It often lasts for a few days and can result in dehydration due to fluid loss. Signs of dehydration often begin with the loss of the normal elasticity of the skin and irritable behaviour. This can progress to decreased urination, loss of skin colour, a fast heart rate, and a decrease in responsiveness as it becomes more severe. Loose but non-watery stools in babies who are exclusively breastfed, however, are normal.

The three types of diarrhoea are: short duration watery diarrhoea, short duration bloody diarrhoea, and persistent diarrhoea (lasting more than two weeks). The short duration watery diarrhoea may be due to an infection by cholera, although this is rare in the developed world. If blood is present, it is also known as dysentery. A number of non-infectious causes can result in diarrhoea. These include lactose intolerance, irritable bowel syndrome, non-celiac gluten sensitivity, celiac disease, inflammatory bowel disease, hyperthyroidism, bile acid diarrhoea, and a number of medications. In most cases, stool cultures to confirm the exact cause are not required.

Acute diarrhoea is most commonly due to viral gastroenteritis with rotavirus, which accounts for 40% of cases in children under five. In travelers, however, bacterial infections predominate. Various toxins such as mushroom poisoning and drugs can also cause acute diarrhoea. Chronic diarrhoea can be part of the presentations of a number of chronic medical conditions affecting the intestine. Common causes include ulcerative colitis, Crohn's disease, microscopic colitis, celiac disease, irritable bowel syndrome and bile acid malabsorption.

Oral rehydration solution (ORS)—clean water with modest amounts of salts and sugar— is the treatment of choice. Zinc tablets are also recommended. These treatments have been estimated to have saved 50 million children in the past 25 years. When people have diarrhoea, it is recommended that they continue to eat healthy food and babies continue to be breastfed. If commercial ORS are not available, homemade solutions may be used. For those with severe dehydration, intravenous fluids may be required. Most cases, however, can be managed well with fluids by mouth. Antibiotics, while rarely used, may be recommended in a few cases such as having bloody diarrhoea and a high fever, having severe diarrhoea following traveling, and growing specific bacteria or parasites in their stool. Loperamide may help decrease the number of bowel movements but is not recommended for those with severe diseases.

🎧 Key Words

elasticity / ˌiːlæˈstɪsəti / n. 弹性

irritable / ˈɪrɪtəbl / adj. 过敏的

responsiveness / rɪˈspɒnsɪvnəs / n. 反应性

exclusively / ɪkˈskluːsɪvli / adv. 唯一地；
专有地

cholera / ˈkɒlərə / n. 霍乱

dysentery / ˈdɪsəntri / n. 痢疾

lactose / ˈlæktəʊs / n. 乳糖

celiac / ˈsiːliæk / adj. 腹腔的

gluten / ˈɡluːtn / n. 谷蛋白

hyperthyroidism / ˌhaɪpəˈθaɪrɔɪdɪzəm / n.
甲状腺功能亢进

rotavirus / ˌrəʊtəˈvaɪərəs / n. 轮状病毒

predominate / prɪˈdɒmɪneɪt / vi.（数量等）占优势

presentation / ˌpreznˈteɪʃn / n. 表现

ulcerative / ˈʌlsərətɪv / adj. 溃疡性的

colitis / kəˈlaɪtɪs / n. 结肠炎

microscopic / ˌmaɪkrəˈskɒpɪk / adj. 用显微镜可见的

malabsorption / ˌmæləbˈzɔːpʃn / n. 吸收不良

loperamide / ˈləʊpərəmaɪd / n. 洛哌丁胺

Useful Expressions

irritable bowel syndrome	肠易激综合征	ulcerative colitis	溃疡性结肠炎
non-celiac gluten sensitivity	非腹腔谷蛋白敏感性	Crohn's disease	克罗恩病，节段性回肠炎
bile acid diarrhoea	胆汁酸性腹泻	oral rehydration solution (ORS)	口服补液

Exercise

I Choose the best answer to each question based on the text.

1. Which of the following is NOT true according to the text? _____.

    A. Diarrhoea can result in dehydration due to fluid loss

    B. Dehydration can cause decreased urination, loss of skin colour, a fast heart rate

    C. Loose but non-watery stools are abnormal for babies who are solely breastfed

2. _____ will last more than two weeks.

    A. Short duration watery diarrhoea

    B. Short duration bloody diarrhoea

    C. Persistent diarrhoea

3. A number of non-infectious causes can result in diarrhoea except _____.

    A. inflammatory bowel disease

    B. dextrose intolerance

    C. irritable bowel syndrome

4. According to Paragraph 3, which of the following is NOT true? _____.

    A. Acute diarrhoea is most commonly due to viral gastroenteritis with rotavirus

    B. Common causes of chronic diarrhoea include ulcerative colitis

    C. Mushroom poisoning and drugs can not cause acute diarrhoea

5. When people have diarrhoea, _____.

    A. intravenous fluids with antibiotics may be required

    B. oral rehydration solution and zinc tablets could be chosen

    C. they are not recommended to continue to eat healthy food

II Match each medical term in Column A with its explanation in Column B.

	Column A	Column B
_____	1. dehydration	a. the fact of not being able to eat particular foods, use particular medicines, etc. without becoming ill
_____	2. intolerance	b. abnormal absorption of nutrients from the digestive tract
_____	3. ulcerative	c. dryness resulting from the removal of water
_____	4. malabsorption	d. characterized by ulceration
_____	5. loperamide	e. a drug which can decrease the number of bowel movements

III Find words or terms in the article to match the following definitions.

1. the condition of having at least three liquid bowel movements each day _____

2. an acute intestinal infection caused by ingestion of contaminated water _____

3. a condition in which the thyroid is too active _____

4. inflammation of the colon _____

IV Critical thinking.

According to the case at the beginning of this unit, what are the nursing diagnoses and the nursing interventions for the patient?

1. Nursing diagnoses

- Fluid volume deficit related to frequent bowel movements
- Hyperthermia related to bacterial or viral infection
- Altered nutrition: less than body requirements related to diarrhoea

2. Nursing interventions

Provision of adequate fluid intake is important in preventing dehydration. IV fluids increase the circulation volume and maintain the fluid and electrolytes balance. Meanwhile the nurse should closely monitor and record the vital signs, skin elasticity, daily weights, intake and output. Increased temperature often indicates the presence of infection or inflammation. It is necessary to send some stool sample to the laboratory.

Part 4 Supplementary Reading

🎧 Electrolytes

An electrolyte is a substance that produces an electrically conducting solution when dissolved in a polar solvent, such as water. The dissolved electrolyte separates into cations and anions, which disperse uniformly through the solvent. Electrically, such a solution is neutral. If an electric potential is applied to such a solution, the cations of the solution are drawn to the electrode that has an abundance of electrons, while the anions are drawn to the electrode that has a deficit of electrons. The movement of anions and cations in opposite directions within the solution amounts to a current.

This includes most soluble salts, acids and bases. Some gases, such as hydrogen chloride, under conditions of high temperature or low pressure can also function as electrolytes. Electrolyte solutions can also result from the dissolution of some biological (e.g., DNA, polypeptides) and synthetic polymers (e.g., polystyrene sulfonate), termed "polyelectrolytes", which contain charged functional groups. A substance that dissociates into ions in solution acquires the capacity to conduct electricity. Sodium, potassium, chloride, calcium, magnesium, and phosphate are examples of electrolytes, informally known as "lytes".

Electrolytes are important, because they are what cells (especially nerve, heart and muscle cells) use to maintain voltages across their cell membranes and to carry electrical impulses (nerve impulses, muscle contractions) across themselves and to other cells. Kidneys work to keep the electrolyte concentrations in blood constant despite changes in the body. For example, during heavy exercise, electrolytes are lost in sweat, particularly in the form of sodium and potassium. These electrolytes must be replaced to keep the electrolyte concentrations of the body fluids constant.

Electrolyte imbalance is an abnormality in the concentration of electrolytes in the body. Electrolytes play a vital role in maintaining homeostasis within the body. They help to regulate heart and neurological function, fluid balance, oxygen delivery, acid–base balance and much more. Electrolyte imbalances can develop by the following mechanisms: excessive ingestion, diminished elimination of an electrolyte, diminished ingestion or excessive elimination of an electrolyte.

The most serious electrolyte disturbances involve abnormalities in the levels of sodium, potassium or calcium. Other electrolyte imbalances are less common, and often occur in conjunction with major electrolyte changes. Chronic laxative abuse or severe diarrhoea or vomiting (gastroenteritis) can lead to electrolyte disturbances along with dehydration. People suffering from bulimia or anorexia nervosa are at especially high risk for an electrolyte imbalance.

Exercise

Choose the best answer to each question based on the text.

1. Which of the following statements is true according to Paragraph 1? _____.

    A. An electrolyte can dissolve in a polar solvent, such as water

    B. A solution which disperses uniformly through the solvent is acidic electrically

    C. The movement of anions and cations in the same direction amounts to a current

2. Electrolyte solutions can NOT result from _____.

    A. ions such as sodium, potassium, chloride

    B. insoluble salts

    C. the dissolution of some biological and synthetic polymers

3. Electrolytes are important, because they can _____.

    A. maintain voltages across the cell membranes

    B. keep the electrolyte concentrations in blood

    C. block electrical impulses across cells and to other cells

4. Electrolyte imbalances can develop by the following mechanisms except _____.

    A. excessive ingestion of an electrolyte

    B. diminished elimination of an electrolyte

    C. excessive ingestion and excessive elimination of an electrolyte

5. Electrolyte disturbances along with dehydration can be led to by _____.

    A. normality in the levels of sodium, potassium or calcium

    B. chronic laxative abuse

    C. mild diarrhoea or vomiting

Part 5 Medical Word Elements

1. esophag(o)-   食管
   esophagoplasty / iˈsɒfəgəˌplæsti /   食管成形术
   esophagoscope / iˈsɒfəgəskəup /   食管镜

2. enter(o)-   小肠
   enterovirus / ˌentərəuˈvaɪərəs /   肠道病毒
   enterostomy / ˌenteˈrɒstəmi /   肠造口术

3. col(o)-   结肠
   colorectal / ˌkəuləˈrektəl /   结肠直肠的
   colonoscope / kəˈlɒnəskəup /   结肠镜检查

4. rect(o)-   直肠
   rectocele / ˈrektəusɪl /   脱肛
   rectopexy / ˈrektəuˌpeksi /   直肠固定术

5. peritone(o)-   腹膜
   peritoneocentesis / ˌperɪˌtəuniəusenˈtiːsɪs /   腹腔穿刺术
   peritoneopathy / ˌperɪtəunɪˈɒpəθi /   腹膜病

6. appendic(o)-   阑尾
   appendicectomy / əˌpendɪˈsektəmi /   阑尾切除术
   appendicitis / əˌpendəˈsaɪtɪs /   阑尾炎

7. ile(o)-   回肠
   ileitis / ˌɪlɪˈaɪtɪs /   回肠炎
   ileorrhaphy / ˌɪlɪˈɒrəfi /   回肠缝合术

8. jejun(o)-   空肠
   jejunostomy / dʒɪdʒuːˈnɒstəmi /   空肠造口术
   jejunum / dʒɪˈdʒuːnəm /   空肠

9. ventr(o)-   腹，前
   ventrolateral / ˌventrəuˈlætərəl /   腹外侧的
   ventrodorsal / ˌventrəuˈdɔːsəl /   腹背（侧）的

（罗晓冰　赵　静）

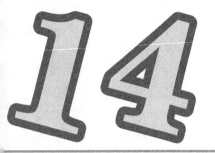

Caring for a Patient with Chronic Obstructive Pulmonary Disease (COPD)

Learning Objectives:

1. *Educating a patient with COPD*
2. *Describing the use of a nebulizer*
3. *Defining and classifying the types of COPD*
4. *Explaining the importance of self-management in COPD care*

Lead-In

Case Study

A 35-year-old man has smoked since he was 18. For the past 3-4 months, he has noticed a mild occasionally productive cough. The cough is worse whenever he spends the night out in the club exposing himself to loads of second-hand smoking. He finally visits his family physician who finds out that he has been smoking about one pack per day. The cough has been on and off for almost a year. He has had no fever or chills. He does admit to more shortness of breath when he exercises over the past six years.

Part 1　Dialogue

🎧 Educating a Patient with COPD

Sue, a ward nurse, is talking about the lifestyle changes with Mr. Smith, a patient, who has been admitted to the hospital for the treatment of COPD again.

Sue:　　　　Good morning, Mr. Smith. I'm glad to see you again.

Mr. Smith:　Good morning, Sue.

Sue:　　　　Are you feeling better today?

Mr. Smith:　I have a feeling of shortness of breath, and I'm coughing seriously.

Sue:　　　　Have you been smoking recently?

Mr. Smith: Yeah, I'm a regular smoker.

Sue: I think this is the problem. Smoking is the primary risk factor for COPD. For you, it is caused by years of smoking. You will have to make some changes in your lifestyle if you're going to avoid complications of COPD.

Mr. Smith: Well, it is difficult for me to give up smoking, but I'll try to do it.

Sue: Very good. I have already taught you several methods to improve the pulmonary function. Could you try to practice some of them in your daily life? Such as breathing exercise, pursed lip breathing or abdominal breathing training, as we know breathing exercise can improve the pulmonary function.

Mr. Smith: All right, I'll make an effort to do that. Anything else should I do?

Sue: Well, what kind of exercise do you usually do?

Mr. Smith: I used to run in the morning, but I haven't been exercising lately.

Sue: Could you try to focus on some cardiovascular exercise in your daily routine? I know it's difficult to exercise when you have trouble breathing, but it can significantly improve the overall strength and endurance of your respiratory muscles.

Mr. Smith: Oh, all right. Mm, what are counted as cardiovascular exercises ?

Sue: Such as biking, brisk walking, jogging, stair climbing are good choices for you.

Mr. Smith: OK, I'll try to do that. Sue, I feel my throat congested with sputum, but sometimes I can't spit it out. What should I do?

Sue: It's difficult to clear your throat but try your best and drink a lot of water every day. If the symptoms persist, please tell me and I will take suction for you.

Mr. Smith: OK, I will do my best. Anything else?

Sue: Pay attention to your symptoms. If the symptoms worsen, please contact us immediately.

Mr. Smith: Thanks. I'll keep that in mind.

Key Words

pulmonary /ˈpʌlmənəri/ *adj.* 肺的
purse /pɜːs/ *v.* 缩拢；噘起
brisk /brɪsk/ *adj.* 轻快的
congest /kənˈdʒest/ *v.* 充满
symptom /ˈsɪmptəm/ *n.* 症状

Useful Expressions

chronic obstructive pulmonary disease (COPD) 慢性阻塞性肺病
short of breath 呼吸短促
regular smoker 经常吸烟者
pulmonary function 肺功能
abdominal breathing 腹式呼吸

Exercise

I **Read the dialogue again and decide whether the following statements are right or wrong. If there is not enough information to answer "Right" or "Wrong", choose "Doesn't say".**

1. The nurse is talking with Mr. Smith about COPD management. _____.

   A. Right　　　　　　B. Wrong　　　　　　C. Doesn't say

2. Mr. Smith has a good control of his smoking. _____.

   A. Right　　　　　　B. Wrong　　　　　　C. Doesn't say

3. Breathing exercise can improve the pulmonary function. _____.

   A. Right　　　　　　B. Wrong　　　　　　C. Doesn't say

4. Cardiovascular exercise can NOT improve the overall strength and the endurance of the patient's respiratory muscles. _____.

   A. Right　　　　　　B. Wrong　　　　　　C. Doesn't say

5. If the symptoms of COPD worsen, the patient should contact medical workers. _____.

   A. Right　　　　　　B. Wrong　　　　　　C. Doesn't say

II **Discussion.**

What significant changes should Mr. Smith make to his lifestyle?

Part 2 Short Passage

🎧 Using a Nebulizer

A nebulizer (or nebuliser) is a drug delivery device used to administer medication in the form of a mist inhaled into the lungs. The nebulizer is composed of four main parts. The first part is a machine. The nebulizer is usually connected to the machine that pushes air through the nebulizer and the air helps turn the medicine into mist. The second part is a tube that acts as a connection between the machine and the medicine cup. The third part is the medicine cup and in it, the medicine is transformed into mist. The fourth part is a mask or mouthpiece that has to be used to breathe the mist in.

Nebulizers are commonly used for the treatment of chronic respiratory diseases, such as asthma and chronic obstructive pulmonary disease (COPD), lung infections, such as pneumonia as well as severe allergic reactions. Nebulizers have a lot of advantages.

1. Nebulizers can be used by anyone of any age.

2. Most nebulizers are small, so they are easy to transport.

3. More than one medicine can be mixed and given at the same time.

4. Nebulizers can deliver medicine with less effort and more effective than other devices.

To use the nebulizer properly, one should follow the steps given below.

1. Wash the hands with soap and water before preparing the nebulizer for use.

2. Fill the chamber of the nebulizer with inhalant medication. Unscrew the top of the nebulizer cup and put the prescribed medication into the nebulizer.

3. Attach the tubing to the machine properly or to the oxygen outlet on the wall.

4. Put on the mask and tighten the elastic straps so that it fits snugly around the head.

5. Turn on the oxygen so the liquid medication turns into a fine mist. Keep medicine container in an upright position.

6. Inhale the mist until it's finished. This takes 10 to 15 minutes. Small children usually do better if they wear a mask.

7. Turn off the machine or the oxygen outlet on the wall when done.

8. Wash the medicine cup and mouthpiece with water and air dry until the next treatment.

🎧 Key Words

inhale / ɪnˈheɪl / v. 吸入，吸气
transform / trænsˈfɔːm / v. 改变，转化
mist / mɪst / n.（药剂的）喷雾

chronic / ˈkrɒnɪk / adj. 慢性的
snugly / ˈsnʌgli / adv. 紧贴地

Useful Expressions

administer medication   用药
respiratory diseases   呼吸系统疾病

allergic reaction   过敏反应
keep sth. in a… position   将某物保持在某一位置

Exercise

I **Choose the best answer to each question based on the text.**

1. A nebulizer is composed of a machine, a tube, a medicine cup and a _____.

   A. line　　　　　B. device　　　　　C. mask

2. Which of the following is the advantage of nebulizers? _____.

   A. It is cheap

   B. It is easy to transport

   C. It needs power supply to function

3. Before preparing the nebulizer for use, one should _____.

   A. wash hands　　　B. put on the mask　　　C. turn on the oxygen

4. Turn on the oxygen so the liquid _____ turns into a fine mist.

   A. water　　　　　B. medication　　　　　C. mist

5. To make sure small children can better use the nebulizer, the best way is to have them_____.

   A. take a machine　　B. carry a cup　　　C. wear a mask

II **Read the passage again and put the following extracts in the correct order.**

   ☐ **A** Breathe in the mist.

   ☐ **B** Turn on the oxygen.

☐ **C** Put on the mask.

☐ **D** Put in the medication.

☐ **E** Connect to the oxygen.

☐ **F** Wash your hands.

Part 3 Text

🎧 Chronic Obstructive Pulmonary Disease

Chronic obstructive pulmonary disease (COPD) is a broad term used to describe conditions characterized by a chronic obstruction to expiratory airflow. Patients with COPD have difficulty emptying their lungs when asked to rapidly and forcefully exhale. COPD is a chronic, progressive disease, meaning it typically worsens over time. Emphysema and chronic bronchitis are the two terms used for different types of COPD.

For most patients, the onset of symptoms is insidious. The most common symptoms of COPD are sputum production, shortness of breath, and a productive cough. These symptoms are present for a prolonged period of time and typically worsen over time. Eventually dyspepsia becomes severe, which forces patients to reduce their level of activity. Patients with COPD gradually become physically disabled. Even everyday activities, such as walking and performing tasks of home maintenance, become difficult.

Most cases of COPD can be prevented by decreasing rates of smoking and improving indoor and outdoor air quality. The effective methods for its treatment include stopping smoking, vaccinations, respiratory rehabilitation, and often inhaled bronchodilators and steroids. Some people may benefit from long-term oxygen therapy or lung transplantation. In those who have periods of acute worsening, increased use of medications and hospitalization may be needed.

Specific lifestyle changes and medical management should be taken seriously. It is necessary to make lifestyle changes. First, stopping smoking is the best preventative measure people can take in avoiding COPD. Second, avoid long-term exposure to irritating fumes, chemicals and air pollution. Third, focus on cardiovascular exercise. Although it's difficult to exercise when people have trouble breathing, it can significantly improve the overall strength and endurance of their respiratory muscles. Building up lung strength through cardiovascular exercises helps lung tissue expand and contract better, which makes breathing and exchanging gases (oxygen for carbon dioxide) more efficient. Then, perform specific breathing exercise. There are two types of breathing patterns that can help promote deeper inhalation/exhalation and provide more comfort: diaphragmatic breathing and pursed-lip breathing. Last, clear the obstructed airways. Mucus is produced by goblet cells in the mucus membranes of the bronchi and other lung tissues in response to chemicals and irritants—people's bodies try to trap and get rid of them; however, the excess mucus collects in their bronchial tubes and contributes to breathing problems. Mucus can be difficult to clear, but clearing one's throat, using a humidifier and drinking lots of water can help get rid of it.

Seeking medical treatment is another important part of COPD management plan. Inhaled bronchodilators, the primary medications, contribute to the overall benefits, such as the relief of breath shortness and wheeze as well as the breakthrough of sports limitation. Consequently, the life quality will be improved overall benefit. They reduce shortness of breath, wheeze, and exercise limitation, resulting in an improved quality of life. Inhaled corticosteroid drugs can quickly reduce airway inflammation and help combat shortness of breath and wheezing associated with COPD. Supplemental oxygen is recommended for those with low oxygen levels at rest.

🎧 Key Words

expiratory / ɪkˈspaɪərətəri / *adj.* 呼气的，吐气的
emphysema / ˌemfɪˈsiːmə / *n.* 肺气肿
insidious / ɪnˈsɪdiəs / *adj.* 隐伏的，潜伏的
dyspepsia / dɪsˈpepsiə / *n.* 消化不良
vaccination / ˌvæksɪˈneɪʃn / *n.* 接种疫苗
bronchodilator / ˌbrɒŋkəʊdaɪˈleɪtə / *n.* 支气管扩张剂

steroid / ˈstɪərɔɪd / *n.* 类固醇
diaphragmatic / ˌdaɪəfrægˈmætɪk / *adj.* 隔膜的
membrane / ˈmembreɪn / *n.* 膜
humidifier / hjuːˈmɪdɪfaɪə(r) / *n.* 增湿器
wheeze / wiːz / *v./n.* 喘息
corticosteroid / ˌkɔːtɪkəʊˈstɪərɔɪd / *n.* 皮质类固醇

Useful Expressions

chronic bronchitis　慢性支气管炎
irritating fumes　刺激性气味

goblet cell　杯状细胞
contribute to　有助于，促成

Exercise

I　Choose the best answer to each question based on the text.

1. How many types of COPD does the text mention? _____.

  A. 1　　　　　　　　B. 2　　　　　　　　C. 3

2. Which one of the following is NOT the symptom of COPD? _____.

  A. A productive cough　　　　　　　B. Shortness of breath

  C. Weight loss

3. Which of the following is the primary risk factor for COPD? _____.

  A. Tobacco smoking　　B. Family history　　　C. Poverty

4. The following are effective ways to control COPD except _____.

  A. giving up smoking　　　　　　　B. performing breathing exercise

  C. lying in bed

5. The following are some medications for COPD except _____.

  A. bronchodilators　　　　　　　　B. tranquilizers

  C. corticosteroids

II　Match each medical term in Column A with its explanation in Column B.

	Column A	Column B
_____	1. COPD	a. a disease that is caused by difficulties in digesting food

	2. dyspepsia	b. relating to the heart and blood vessels
	3. sputum	c. a thin piece of skin that connects parts of one's body
	4. cardiovascular	d. wet substance coughed up from one's lung
	5. membrane	e. a disease that causes difficulties in breathing

III **Find words or terms in the article to match the following definitions.**

1. It is one type of COPD that occurs when the lungs become larger and do NOT work properly, causing difficulty in breathing _____

2. It is one type of COPD that occurs when the inflamed bronchial tubes produce a lot of mucus, leading to coughing and difficulty in breathing _____

3. any drug that causes dilation of the bronchial tubes by relaxing bronchial muscle _____

4. the process or act of breathing in, taking air and sometimes other substances into one's lungs _____

IV **Critical thinking.**

According to the case at the beginning of this unit, what are the nursing diagnoses and the nursing interventions for the patient?

1. Nursing diagnoses

   • Ineffective airway clearance related to increased secretions and ineffective cough

   • Ineffective breathing patterns related to altered pulmonary mechanics

   • Activity intolerance related to decreased oxygen delivery to tissues

2. Nursing interventions

   To reduce airway resistance the nurse administers antibiotics, bronchodilators and steroids as ordered by the physician. Interventions to improve airway clearance include deep breathing and coughing techniques. The administration of oxygen by nasal cannula should be sufficient to maintain adequate SaO_2. Meanwhile patient should limit physical activities to reduce oxygen consumption.

Part 4 Supplementary Reading

🎧 Sputum Suction

Sputum suction is the process of removing the secretions that patients can not remove through coughing. The purposes of sputum suction are to maintain the patient's airway patent and prevent the patient's airway obstructions, to promote the patient's respiratory function (optimal exchange of oxygen and carbon dioxide into and out of the lungs) as well as to prevent pneumonia that may results from accumulated secretions.

Sputum suction should be done when secretions have accumulated or adventitious breath sounds are audible. Depending on the patient's condition, sputum suction can be used in different ways of oropharyngeal, nasopharyngeal, nasotracheal and endotracheal or tracheal tube. The suction of the nose and mouth is a relatively simple procedure requiring only cleanliness and sensible care in the removal of liquids obstructing the nasal and oral passages. The Suction of the deeper respiratory structures demands special skill and meticulous care to avoid traumatizing the delicate mucous membrane and introducing infection into the respiratory tract.

Before the suction, the nurse should assess the patient's understanding of the procedure of the suction, and explain to the patient that the suction will relieve the breathing difficulty and that the procedure is painless but may be uncomfortable and stimulate the cough, gag, or sneeze reflex. Meanwhile, the nurse should encourage the patient to cooperate and relax. There are two different positions when the nurse takes suction. One is to position a conscious patient who has a functional gag reflex in the semi-Fowler's position with head turned to one side for the oral suction or with neck hyper-extended for the nasal suction. This position facilitates the insertion of the catheter and helps prevent the aspiration of secretions. The other is to position an unconscious patient in the lateral position, facing the nurse. This position allows the tongue to fall forward, so that it will not obstruct the catheter during the insertion. This position also makes easier the drainage of secretions from the pharynx and prevents the possibility of aspiration.

When suctioning, set the negative pressure on the suction gauge (Adults: 300-400 mmHg; Children: 250-300 mmHg). Open the suction catheter by using the aseptic technique, open the sterile basin and place it on the bedside table, and then pour about 100 mL sterile water or normal saline into the basin. With the sterile gloved hand, pick up the sterile catheter and connect it to the suction tubing, and suck a small amount of normal saline from the basin, finally suck the airway. The nurse should record the time of suction and the nature and amount of the secretions. Note the character of the client's respiratory before and after the suction.

Exercise

Choose the best answer to each question based on the text.

1. The purposes of the sputum suction are the following except _____.
   A. maintaining the patient's airway patent
   B. preventing the airway obstructions
   C. treating pneumonia

2. Which of the following statements is NOT true according to the passage? _____.
   A. Sputum suction is the process of removing the secretions that patients can not remove through coughing
   B. One of the purposes of the sputum suction is to promote the patient's respiratory function
   C. Sputum suction can be done by anyone

3. What is the advantage of the sputum suction? _____.
   A. Breathing difficulty will be relieved   B. The procedure is comfortable
   C. Cough, gag or sneeze reflex will be relieved

4. When suctioning, the nurse should make sure _____.
   A. the aseptic technique is employed   B. the patient feels relaxed
   C. the patient lies in bed

5. Which of the following statements is true according to the passage? _____.

   A. When suctioning for children, the nurse should set the negative pressure on the suction gauge at 300 - 400 mmHg

   B. The nurse should note the character of the client's respiratory before and after suctioning

   C. Being sterile is not very important during the operation of suction

Part 5 Medical Word Elements

1. carb(o)-   碳
   carbhemoglobin / ˌkɑːbhɪməʊˈgləʊbɪn /   碳酸血红蛋白
   carbohydrate / ˌkɑːbəʊˈhaɪdreɪt /   碳水化合物
2. pulmon(o)-   肺
   pulmonology / ˌpʌlməˈnɒlədʒi /   肺脏病学
   cardiopulmonary / ˌkɑːdiəʊˈpʌlmənəri /   心肺的
3. pleur(o)-   胸膜
   pleurocentesis / ˌpluərəʊsenˈtiːsɪs /   胸腔穿刺术
   pleurodynia / ˌpluərəʊˈdɪniə /   胸膜痛
4. ket(o)-   酮（基）
   ketoacidemia / ˌkiːtəʊˌæsɪˈdiːmiə /   酮酸血症
   ketoacidosis / ˌkiːtəʊˌæsɪˈdəʊsɪs /   酮酸中毒
5. adren(o)-   肾上腺
   adrenoceptor / æˌdriːnəʊˈseptə /   肾上腺素能受体
   adrenocortical / əˌdriːnəʊˈkɔːtɪkl /   肾上腺皮质的
6. tonsill(o)-   扁桃体
   tonsillitis / ˌtɒnsəˈlaɪtɪs /   扁桃体炎
   tonsillotomy / ˌtɒnsiˈlɒtəmi /   扁桃体切除术
7. di-   二，双
   dioxide / daɪˈɒksaɪd /   二氧化物
   dioxygenase / daɪˈɒksɪˌdʒeneɪs /   双加氧酶
8. -meter   计、表、量器
   cephalometer / ˌsefəˈlɒmɪtə /   头部测量器
   thermometer / θəˈmɒmɪtə(r) /   温度计
9. -megaly   异常扩大
   cardiomegaly / ˌkɑːdiəʊˈmegəli /   心脏扩大症
   chiromegaly / ˌkaɪrəˈmegəli /   巨手

（宋洪玲　赵　静）

Caring for a Patient with Hip Replacement

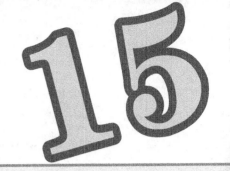

Learning Objectives:

1. *Describing the steps of transporting patients from bed to chair*
2. *Describing the steps of transporting patients from chair to bed*
3. *Defining and classifying the different types of hip replacement and explaining some tips for making the patient's life easier*
4. *Discussing the preparations a patient should make before he or she goes for the physical therapy*

Lead-In

Case Study

A 35-year-old female patient was referred with pains on the right side of pelvis. She was investigated for back and hip problems. All her blood results including inflammatory markers were normal. Radiographs and bone scan were normal. She was thought to have hip dysplasia and a MRI revealed abnormal signal changes in the right ilium suggestive of neoplasia or infection. She was afebrile and had no history of infections and exposure to tuberculosis.

Part 1 Dialogue

🎧 Talking with a Patient About Falling

Mr. Brown fell on his left shoulder and left leg when he went downstairs this afternoon. He called Dr. Lee immediately to make an appointment. When he arrived, Dr. Lee was having a patient. Dr. Lee's nurse Lucy gave him a warm reception first.

Lucy:　　　　Hello, Mr. Brown. Dr. Lee is having a patient inside now, but it won't take too long. Wait here for a moment. Do you need some drinks?

Mr. Brown:　No, thank you, Lucy. It's very kind of you.

Lucy:　　　　How did it happen?

Mr. Brown:　When I went downstairs this afternoon, I fell on my left shoulder and left leg.

Lucy:	They look black and blue now. You must be painful.
Mr. Brown:	Not really. Sometimes I feel numb in it.
Lucy:	Have you taken any painkillers?
Mr. Brown:	Not yet.
Lucy:	Can you move your left arm and your left leg?
Mr. Brown:	I can't move them. Do you think it's normal?
Lucy:	I am not sure, but you don't need to worry about it. You know, Dr. Lee is excellent in this field. Mr. Brown, Dr. Lee is available now. This way, please.
Mr. Brown:	Thank you.

(After Dr. Lee's examination and treatment…)

Lucy:	Do you feel better?
Mr. Brown:	Of course. I can move my left arm freely after the relocation, but I can't move my left leg.
Lucy:	The X-ray picture shows your left shoulder is dislocated. Dr. Lee has already relocated it. The external form of your left shoulder has been restored normally. Unluckily, you have a displaced fracture of the tibia and fibula. It's a little troublesome. You need to stay in bed for at least one month. Dr. Lee has put the plaster on you.
Mr. Brown:	A month? It is too long for me. I will go on a business trip next week.
Lucy:	You'd better cancel it, because you should have a good rest in bed. You know, if the reduction of the fracture is unsatisfactory, the procedure of course must be repeated. It will be more painful.
Mr. Brown:	Sounds terrible. When can I walk?
Lucy:	Dr. Lee just told you during these early weeks you should take regular X-ray to make sure that the reduction is maintained. And then he will tell you when you are able to walk. Just be patient. Don't forget to take pills on time and lift your left leg on a pillow when you are lying.
Mr. Brown:	You are very thoughtful. Thank you.
Lucy:	My pleasure.

🎧 Key Words

painkiller / ˈpeɪnkɪlə(r) / *n.* 止痛药

dislocate / ˈdɪsləkeɪt / *v.* 脱臼

relocate / riːləʊˈkeɪt / *v.* 重新定位；复位

external / ɪkˈstɜːnl / *adj.* 外部的；表面的

restore / rɪˈstɔː(r)/ *v.* 恢复；修复

tibia / ˈtɪbiə / *n.* 胫骨

fibula / ˈfɪbjələ / *n.* 腓骨

plaster / ˈplɑːstə/ *n.* 石膏

reduction / rɪˈdʌkʃn / *n.* 复位

Useful Expressions

black and blue　青肿的；淤血的　　　　displaced fracture　移位性骨折
be available　有空

Exercise

1 **Read the dialogue again and decide whether the following statements are right or wrong. If there is not enough information to answer "Right" or "Wrong", choose "Doesn't say".**

1. Mr. Brown hurt his shoulders and legs when he went downstairs this afternoon. _____.

　　A. Right　　　　　　B. Wrong　　　　　C. Doesn't say

2. Mr. Brown's left arm needs relocating. _____.

　　A. Right　　　　　　B. Wrong　　　　　C. Doesn't say

3. Mr. Brown wears the plaster because of a displaced fracture of the left arm. _____.

　　A. Right　　　　　　B. Wrong　　　　　C. Doesn't say

4. Accompanied by the nurse, Mr. Brown has an X-ray. _____.

　　A. Right　　　　　　B. Wrong　　　　　C. Doesn't say

5. As soon as the X-ray shows the reduction is maintained, Mr. Brown can walk. _____.

　　A. Right　　　　　　B. Wrong　　　　　C. Doesn't say

2 **Discussion.**

Imagine the process of Dr. Lee's treatment and tell what matters Mr. Brown should pay attention to.

Part 2 Short Passage

🎧 Transporting a Patient on a Wheelchair

　　The safe transporting of patients is different from industrial load transporting. Industrial load can be packaged to provide easier positioning for manual handling, or can be transferred by mechanical lifters. In contrast, the patient can be easily hurt by improper transporting. In addition, the comfort of the patients and the safety of the nurses should also be considered. A lot of nurses will injure their backs through patient transporting. To do this effectively, nurses must master the knowledge of transporting procedures. For this reason the procedures are presented below.

　　1. Put the chair or the wheelchair next to the bed on the patient's strong side, if the patient has a weak side. It can reduce the risk of falling and the nurse's load.

　　2. Bring the patient into a sitting position at the side of the bed, which can enable the patient to participate as much as possible.

　　3. Put the transfer belt around the patient's waist, which provides safe, balanced hold on patients without pressurizing joints or limbs.

　　4. For better stability, the nurse's feet should be wide apart, one foot pointing toward one side

of the bed, the other toward the chair.

5. Support the patient's close knees with the front legs; the nurse's other leg should be back to create a wide base of support.

6. To share part of the load, patient's arms should be put on the nurse's shoulders.

7. The nurse's knees should be well flexed with the back straight, hands gripping each side of the transfer belt. Remember to use the thigh muscles to reduce the back strain.

8. Coordinate the efforts of the nurse and the patient; use of the thighs, arms, and weight of the nurse to move the patient load.

9. The patient should be asked to move his/her leg closest to wheelchair forward (if possible).

10. The nurse should face the chair and the patient's back should face the chair; the nurse should still hold the transfer belt.

11. The patient should reach down and grip armrests; the backs of legs should touch chair.

12. As the patient eases himself/herself into the chair using the armrests for support, the nurse supports one of the patient's knees with his/her own knee and the nurse's feet prevent the patient's foot from sliding forward. Nurse flexes his/her own knees to lower the patient into the chair.

13. As the weakened patient may fall out of the chair, patient should be supported in wheelchair when in need.

To move the patient from the wheelchair to the bed, the entire procedure should be reversed. However, every patient is a unique individual. Although the basic principles of transporting patients are well built, it is necessary to make some changes to meet the needs of the individual patients.

🎧 Key Words

participate / pɑːˈtɪsɪpeɪt / v. 参与，参加	grip / ɡrɪp / v. 紧握
waist / weɪst / n. 腰，腰部	strain / streɪn / n. 张力
joint / dʒɔɪnt / n. 关节	armrest / ˈɑːmrest / n. 扶手；靠手
limb / lɪm / n. 肢，臂	reverse / rɪˈvɜːs / v. 颠倒
flex / fleks / v. 弯曲	

Useful Expressions

in contrast　与此相反	closest to　离……最近
coordinate efforts　齐心协力	basic principles　基本原则

Exercise

1 Choose the best answer to each question based on the text.

1. What should be considered when a patient is transported? ＿＿＿＿.

　　A. The comfort of the patient　　　　B. The safety of the nurse

　　C. Both A and B

2. A nurse should put chair or wheelchair next to the bed on patient's ＿＿＿＿ side during the transporting.

　　A. strong　　　　B. weak　　　　C. any

3. To enable the patient to participate as much as possible, the nurse should bring the patient into a _____position.

    A. standing   B. sitting   C. lying

4. To share part of the load, the patient's arms should be put on _____.

    A. the bed   B. the armrest of the wheelchair

    C. the nurse's shoulders

5. To reduce the back strain, the nurse should _____.

    A. coordinate with the patient

    B. use the thigh muscles

    C. grip the transfer belt

II Read the passage again and put the following extracts in the correct order.

    ☐ **A** Bring the patient into a sitting position at the side of the bed.

    ☐ **B** the patient's arms should be put on the nurse's shoulders.

    ☐ **C** the nurse's feet should be wide apart, using one leg to create a wide base of support.

    ☐ **D** Put the chair or the wheelchair next to the bed on the patient's strong side.

    ☐ **E** The nurse should face the chair and the patient's back should face the chair.

    ☐ **F** Put the transfer belt around the patient's waist.

    ☐ **G** The patient should ease himself/herself into the chair using the armrests for support.

Part 3 Text

🎧 Hip Replacement

Hip replacement is a surgical procedure in which the hip joint is replaced by a prosthetic implant, that is, a hip prosthesis. Hip replacement surgery can be performed as a total replacement which is also called the total hip arthroplasty or hemireplacement that is hemiarthroplasty. The total hip replacement is most commonly used to treat joint failure caused by osteoarthritis, which consists of replacing both the acetabulum and the femoral head. While hemiarthroplasty generally replaces one half of the joint with an artificial surface and leaves the other part in its natural state. If other treatments such as physical therapy, pain killer, and exercise have failed, hip replacement surgery might be the best option.

During the standard hip replacement surgery, the patient is given general anaesthesia to relax muscles and falls into a temporary deep sleep. This will prevent the patient from feeling any pain during the surgery or have any awareness of the procedure. A spinal anaesthesia may be given to help prevent pain as an alternative. The surgeon will then make a cut along the side of the hip and move the muscles connected to the top of the thighbone to expose the hip joint. Next, the ball portion of the joint is removed by cutting the thighbone with a saw. Then an artificial joint using either cement or a special material allows the remaining bone to attach to the new joint. Since there would be some blood loss during the hip replacement surgery, a blood transfusion may be needed.

Therefore, the patient should consider donating his or her own blood before the procedure.

The hip replacement patients typically stay in hospital for 2 to 5 days after the surgery. It is very important for the nurse to pay attention to the complications of the patients. If prompt treatments are not carried out on time, it will harm the patients. The nurse should also be aware of the potential complications which are dislocation of the hip prosthesis, excessive wound drainage, infection and so on. Nursing care plans should focus on preventing the occurrence of the complications.

It takes most patients between 6 weeks to 3 months to stop taking pain medication and regain the ability to walk and do most daily activities. During that time patients may use walking aids such as a cane. Driving or other physical activities should not be permitted without the doctor's approval. Even after the hip joint has been healed, certain sports or heavy activities should be avoided. The replacement joint is designed for usual day-to-day activity.

There are some simple tips that can make the patients' lives easier when they return home after the hip replacement surgery.

- Keep stairs climbing to a minimum, no more than once or twice a day.
- Sit in a firm, straight-back chair.
- Avoid falls.
- Make the toilet seat higher.
- Keep the enthusiastic pets away until the patients have completely recovered.

🎧 Key Words

arthroplasty / ˈɑːθrəˌplæsti / n. 关节成形术；关节造形术
osteoarthritis / ˌɒstɪəʊɑːˈθraɪtɪs / n. 骨关节炎
acetabulum / ˌæsɪˈtæbjʊləm / n. 髋臼；关节窝

artificial / ˌɑːtɪˈfɪʃl / adj. 人造的
spinal / ˈspaɪnl / adj. 脊髓的；脊柱的
thighbone / ˈθaɪbəʊn / n. 股骨；大腿骨

Useful Expressions

hip replacement   髋关节置换
prosthetic implant   假体性植入物
femoral head   股骨头

physical therapy   物理疗法
wound drainage   伤口引流

Exercise

1 Choose the best answer to each question based on the text.

1. Hip replacement consists of _____ and _____.

   A. total hip arthroplasty; hemiarthroplasty

   B. total replacement; hemireplacement

   C. both A and B

2. What does the total hip replacement most commonly treat? _____.

   A. Joint failure   B. Osteoarthritis   C. Osteonecrosis

3. What does the total hip replacement consist of? _____.

   A. Replacing the acetabulum   B. Replacing both the acetabulum and the femoral head

C. Replacing the femoral head

4. What should nursing care plans focus on? _____.

   A. Prompting healing   B. Developing good habits

   C. Preventing the occurrence of the complications

5. Which of the following statements is NOT true according to the passage? _____.

   A. The patient should consider donating his or her own blood before the procedure

   B. The nurse should also be aware of the potential complications

   C. The total hip arthroplasty generally replaces one half of the joint with an artificial surface and leaves the other part in its natural state

Ⅱ Match each medical term in Column A with its explanation in Column B.

Column A	Column B
_____ 1. prosthesis	a. the large bone in the upper part of a human leg
_____ 2. osteoarthritis	b. an artificial body part which takes the place of a missing part
_____ 3. acetabulum	c. chronic breakdown of cartilage in the joints
_____ 4. thighbone	d. a surgical replacement of a degenerated joint
_____ 5. arthroplasty	e. a concave surface of a pelvis

Ⅲ Find words or terms in the article to match the following definitions.

1. a surgical procedure in which the hip joint is replaced by a prosthetic implant _____

2. a surgical operation commonly used to treat joint failure caused by osteoarthritis _____

3. a surgical operation generally used to replace one half of the joint with an artificial surface and leaves the other part in its natural state _____

4. the use of anaesthetics to relax muscles and falls the patient into a temporary deep sleep during the surgery _____

5. a process in which blood is injected into the body of a person who is facing blood loss _____

Ⅳ Critical thinking.

According to the case at the beginning of this unit, what are the nursing diagnoses and the nursing interventions for the patient?

1. Nursing diagnoses

   • Pain, acute, related to surgical procedure or abnormal bone development

   • Impaired physical mobility related to pain or surgical procedure

2. Nursing interventions

Any special equipment that will be used is demonstrated to the patient. The nurse ensures that the patient know how to use the PCA machine and further assists the patient in managing pain by position changes and back care. The incision is monitored for erythema, drainage and any signs of infection. A pillow is placed between the patient's legs after the hip replacement to prevent dislocation.

Part 4 Supplementary Reading

🎧 Physiotherapy

Physical therapy (PT), also known as physiotherapy, is one of the allied health professions. It remediates impairments and promotes mobility and function by using mechanical force and movements (biomechanics or kinesiology), manual therapy, exercise therapy and electrotherapy. It's also used to improve the patient's quality of life through examination, diagnosis, prognosis and physical intervention.

What conditions can physiotherapy treat? It mainly focuses on the restoration and rehabilitation of the circulatory and musculoskeletal systems. It can also be used to treat the conditions such as sports injuries, arthritis and respiratory problems. Therefore, it can treat a variety of health problems including relieving pain, improving movement or ability, preventing or recovering from a sports injury, preventing disability or surgery, working on balance to prevent a slip or fall, managing a chronic illness, recovering after giving birth, adapting to an artificial limb, controlling bowels or bladder, learning to use assistive devices like a walker or cane and so on.

Physical therapy is a professional career which has many specialties. When a patient is preparing for physiotherapy, there are a few things he or she can do in order to have a positive experience. Firstly, ask questions before choosing a physical therapist. Physical therapists are commonly called PTs who work with patients to prevent the loss of mobility before it occurs. They help patients to develop fitness and wellness-oriented programs for healthier and more active lifestyles, providing services to patients to develop, maintain and restore maximum movement and functional ability throughout the lifespan. The overall conditions can be evaluated and assessed by PTs when the patient first visits. PTs may take specific measurements to gather information about the patient's illness or injury. Secondly, PTs will discuss the goals for physical therapy and work with the patient to develop a treatment plan, so the patient should be prepared to tell exactly what he or she hopes to achieve during therapy. If the patient doesn't understand a specific treatment during the PT sessions, ask PTs directly. The relationship between the physical therapist and the patient should feel like an alliance, which can make both of them achieve specific goals.

Exercise

Choose the best answer to each question based on the text.

1. What are the functions of physiotherapy? _____.

    A. To remediate impairments and promote mobility and function

    B. To improve the patient's quality of life

    C. Both A and B

2. Physiotherapy can treat a variety of health problems except _____.

A. sports injuries   B. respiratory problems

C. hypertension in the very elderly

3. When a patient is preparing for physiotherapy, who will evaluate the patient's overall conditions? _____.

A. The surgeon   B. The nurse   C. The physical therapist

4. What's the relationship between the physical therapist and the patient? _____.

A. As alliance   B. As teacher and student

C. As doctor and patient

5. Which of the following statements is NOT true according to the passage? _____.

A. The patient should choose a physical therapist before asking questions

B. Physical therapist will discuss the goals for physiotherapy with the patient

C. Physiotherapy functions by using mechanical force and movements, manual therapy, exercise therapy and electrotherapy

Part 5 Medical Word Elements

1. arthr(o)-	关节
arthroendoscopy / ˌɑːθrəʊenˈdɒskəpi /	关节镜检查
arthrolithiasis / ˌɑːθrəlɪˈθaɪəsɪs /	痛风
2. -plasty	成形术，整形术
dermatoplasty / ˈdɜːmətəʊˌplæsti /	皮肤移植，植皮术
rhinoplasty / ˌraɪnəˈplæsti /	鼻整形术
3. my(o)-	肌
myocarditis / ˌmaɪəʊkɑːˈdaɪtɪs /	心肌炎
myophagism / maɪˈɑfədʒizəm /	肌萎缩
4. chondr(o)-	软骨
chondrocyte / ˈkɒndrəʊsaɪt /	软骨细胞
chondroitin / kɒnˈdrəʊɪtɪn /	软骨素
5. -rrhaphy	缝术，修复术
hepatorrhaphy / ˌhepəˈtɒrəfi /	肝缝合术
myorrhaphy / maɪˈɒrəfi /	肌缝合术
6. peri-	周围，周
pericardium / ˌperɪˈkɑːdiəm /	心包膜
perinatal / ˌperɪˈneɪtl /	围产期的
7. -trophy	营养
myoatrophy / ˌmaɪəʊˈætrəfi /	肌萎缩
neurotrophy / njuəˈrɒtrəfi /	神经营养

8. -oma   瘤

encephaloma /ˌensefəˈləʊmə/   脑瘤

fibroadenoma /ˌfaɪbrəʊˌædɪˈnəʊmə/   纤维腺瘤

9. -rrhagia   出血

metrorrhagia /ˌmiːtrəˈreɪdʒɪə/   子宫不规则出血

rhinorrhagia /ˌraɪnəˈreɪdʒɪə/   鼻出血

（韩亚蕾　赵　静）

Caring for a Pregnant Woman

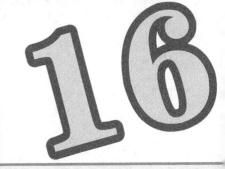

Learning Objectives:

1. *Discussing the correct gesture and way of breastfeeding*
2. *Describing the procedures of the Leopold's manoeuvres*
3. *Defining and classifying the three common types of gestational hypertension*
4. *Explaining the advantages of blue light therapy in treating neonatal jaundice*

Lead-In

Case Study

A 43-year-old woman presented herself to the antenatal day unit at the 32nd weeks' gestation with a blood pressure of 157/93 mmHg. Her first pregnancy was 32. She was a non-smoker and had no known drug allergies. Earlier in the day, she had a headache that was relieved by paracetamol. Urinalysis showed protein (1+) and a urinary protein creatinine ratio of 19 mg/mmol. Further measurements found a blood pressure of 163/96 mmHg. At the 34th weeks' gestation she presented herself to the labour ward with a blood pressure of 158/98 mmHg. Urinary protein creatinine ratio was 39 mg/mmol.

Part 1 Dialogue

🎧 Educating a Patient About Breastfeeding

Mrs. White gave birth to baby yesterday. Nurse Mary visits her this morning. Mary cares about Mrs. White's sleep as well as breastfeeding, and shows her the correct breastfeeding way. As a new mom, Mrs. White asks her some basic questions about feeding and keeping fit. She takes Mary's advice at last.

Mary:	Good morning, Mrs. White. How about your sleep yesterday?
Mrs. White:	Not very well. I am always between wake and sleep.
Mary:	It's normal at the beginning of being a mom. How's the breastfeeding going?
Mrs. White:	The baby's sucking well but I don't have much milk.
Mary:	Don't worry. That will come soon. Make sure that you put the baby's tongue well under your nipple, and then you use one hand to keep the breast in his mouth.

Mrs. White:	How often need I feed my baby?
Mary:	A newborn has a small stomach capacity. During the first few weeks babies may express demand for feeding every one to three hours (8-12 times in 24 hours). Older children feed less often. Sometimes babies may also need nursing when they are lonely, frightened or in pain. So the sucking patterns and needs of babies are different.
Mrs. White:	How long will a feeding take?
Mary:	The duration of feeding is usually ten to fifteen minutes on each breast. But during the newborn period, most breastfeeding sessions take from 20 to 45 minutes. After one breast is empty, you may offer the other breast. Sucking causes the contraction of the uterus. If you feel some cramps in your uterus when you are feeding him, it's normal.
Mrs. White:	How long will exclusive breastfeeding last?
Mary:	Normally speaking I recommend breastfeeding exclusively for six months. This means it is no need to feed the baby other food or drinks except for possibly vitamin D. Your milk can fully meet the nutritional needs of the baby. Even after the introduction of foods at six months of age, I advise you to continue breastfeeding until at least one to two years of age.
Mrs. White:	When can I start to keep on a diet and lose weight?
Mary:	You'd better not keep on a diet when you are feeding your baby. You know your milk is the ideal food for your baby. If you want to keep fit, you should keep a balanced diet and have moderate physical activities. As we all know, breastfeeding has a number of benefits to both mothers and babies including keeping fit.
Mrs. White:	Thank you for your advice. I will follow it.
Mary:	You are welcome. Whenever you have some questions, please ask me any time.

🎧 Key Words

suck / sʌk / v. 吸吮
nipple / 'nɪpl / n. 乳头
newborn / 'njuːbɔːn / adj./n. 新生儿（的）
capacity / kə'pæsəti / n. 容量
duration / dju'reɪʃn /n. 持续的时间

contraction / kən'trækʃn / n. 收缩，紧缩
uterus / 'juːtərəs / n. 子宫
cramp / kræmp / n. 痉挛，绞痛
nutritional / njuˈtrɪʃənl / adj. 营养的；滋养的
breastfeed / 'brestfiːd / vt. 母乳喂养

Useful Expressions

keep on a diet 控制饮食

balanced diet 均衡饮食

Exercise

I **Read the dialogue again and decide whether the following statements are right or wrong. If there is not enough information to answer "Right" or "Wrong", choose "Doesn't say".**

1. Mrs. White had a good sleep yesterday. _____.

   A. Right   B. Wrong   C. Doesn't say

2. Mrs. White has too much milk but her baby doesn't know how to suck. _____.

   A. Right   B. Wrong   C. Doesn't say

3. When babies are hungry, lonely, frightened or in pain, they need to be fed. _____.

   A. Right   B. Wrong   C. Doesn't say

4. Most mothers have exclusively breastfed their babies for six months. _____.

   A. Right   B. Wrong   C. Doesn't say

5. Mrs. White can keep a balanced diet and have moderate physical activities immediately after having a baby. _____.

   A. Right   B. Wrong   C. Doesn't say

II **Discussion.**

Talk about the correct gesture and way of breastfeeding.

Part 2 Short Passage

🎧 Leopold's Manoeuvres

Leopold's manoeuvres, which are named after the gynecologist Christian Gerhard Leopold, are a common way to determine the position and the presentation of a fetus inside the woman's uterus.

The manoeuvres consist of four steps. To perform the manoeuvres, the examiners should first ensure that the woman has recently emptied her bladder. Then let the woman lie on her back with her shoulders raised slightly on a pillow and her knees lifting a little. The woman's abdomen should be uncovered. Try to make the woman feel relaxed and have a right position. If the examiners warm their hands before performing the manoeuvres, most women would appreciate it.

The examiner should explain the procedure and the basic principle for each step to the woman. Tell her what is found at each step.

The first manoeuvre

Palpate the uterine fundus. The breech feels softer and more irregular in shape than the head. Moving the breech will also move the trunk. The head is harder, with a round, regular shape. The head will move without moving the entire trunk.

The second manoeuvre

Hold the left hand steady on one side of the uterus while palpating the opposite of the uterus with the right hand. Then hold the right hand steady while palpating the opposite side of the uterus with the left hand. The fetal back is a smooth convex surface. The fetal arms and legs feel nodular and the fetus will often move them during palpation.

The third manoeuvre

Palpate the suprapubic area. If a breech was palpated in the fundus, expect a hard, rounded head in this area. Attempt to grasp the presenting part gently between the thumb and fingers. If the presenting part is not engaged, the grasping movement of the fingers will easily move it upward in the uterus. If the fetus is in a breech presentation, omit the fourth manoeuvre.

The fourth manoeuvre

The last manoeuvre requires that the examiner faces the woman's feet. The fingers of both hands moves gently down the sides of the uterus. On one side, the examiner's fingers will easily slide to the upper edge of the symphysis. On the other side, the fingers will meet an obstruction.

Leopold's manoeuvres should be performed by health care professionals, as they have received the relative training. If performed at home, the examiner should take care not to disturb the fetus too much.

🎧 Key Words

manoeuvre / məˈnuːvə(r) / n. 手法；操作法
gynecologist / ˌɡaɪnəˈkɒlədʒɪst / n. 妇科医生
fetus / ˈfiːtəs / n. 胎儿
palpate / pælˈpeɪt / v. 触诊
breech / briːtʃ / n. 臀部

fetal / ˈfiːtl / adj. 胎儿的
convex / ˈkɒnveks / adj. 凸圆的
nodular / ˈnɒdjulə / adj. 结节状的；有结节的
suprapubic / ˌsuːprəˈpjuːbɪk / adj. 耻骨弓上的
symphysis / ˈsɪmfəsɪs / n. （骨的）联合；联合线

Useful Expressions

Leopold's manoeuvres 利奥波德（产科）手法（四步触诊法）
uterine fundus   子宫底

convex surface   凸面；背弧面
breech presentation   臀先露

Exercise

1 Choose the best answer to each question based on the text.

1. What's the purpose of performing Leopold's manoeuvres? _____.

   A. To determine the weight of a fetus   B. To determine the delivery way

   C. To determine the position and the presentation of a fetus

2. To perform the manoeuvres, what should the pregnant woman prepare to do? _____.

   A. To empty her stomach

   B. To empty her bladder

   C. To drink some water

3. What should the examiner explain to the pregnant woman when each step is done? _____.

   A. The procedure and the basic principle for each step

   B. What is found at each step

C. Both A and B

4. Fetus's head feels _____ when the examiner performs the first manoeuvre.

　　A. softer and more irregular

　　B. softer and more regular

　　C. harder and more regular

5. When the examiner is palpating the suprapubic area, the _____ of the fetus is expected in this area if a breech was palpated in the fundus.

　　A. head　　　　　　B. breech　　　　　　C. trunk

Ⅱ Read the passage again and put the following extracts in the correct order.

☐ **A** The pregnant woman lies on her back.

☐ **B** The examiner palpates both sides of the uterus.

☐ **C** The pregnant woman empties her bladder.

☐ **D** The examiner palpates the uterine fundus.

☐ **E** The examiner palpates the suprapubic area.

☐ **F** The examiner warms his/her hands.

Part 3　Text

🎧 Pregnancy-Induced Hypertension

　　Pregnancy-induced hypertension (PIH) is also called pre-eclampsia or pregnancy toxemia. It is a pregnancy complication characterized by high blood pressure, swelling due to fluid retention, and protein in the urine. High blood pressure is also called hypertension. Its systolic and diastolic pressures equal to or exceed 140/90 mmHg. PIH develops after the 20th week of pregnancy. This condition can cause serious problems for both the mother and the baby if left untreated.

　　Some pregnant women may have hypertension or swelling, but these conditions don't mean they have PIH. What are the symptoms of pregnancy-induced hypertension? Rapid or sudden weight gain, high blood pressure, protein in the urine, and swelling (in the hands, feet, and face) are all signs of PIH. Some swelling is normal during pregnancy. However, if the swelling doesn't go away and is accompanied by some of the above symptoms, be sure to see a doctor right away. Other symptoms of PIH include abdominal pain, severe headaches, a change in reflexes, spots before your eyes, reduced output of urine or no urine, blood in the urine, dizziness, or excessive vomiting and nausea.

　　Pregnancy-induced hypertension is more common during a woman's first pregnancy and in women whose mothers or sisters had PIH. Although PIH more commonly occurs during first pregnancies, it can also occur in subsequent pregnancies. Women who are carrying multiple babies, in teenage or over the age of 40 will have a higher risk of PIH. Women who had high blood pressure or kidney disease before pregnancy also have a tendency to develops PIH. Generally, PIH occurs during the second half of pregnancy, usually after the 20th week, but it can also develops at the time of delivery or after delivery.

No one test diagnoses PIH. During the routine prenatal tests, the weight gain, blood pressure and urine protein are monitored. If PIH is suspected, a non-stress test may be performed to monitor the baby. During the non-stress test, the baby's heart rate is recorded by an ultrasound transducer, and the uterine activity is recorded by a pressure transducer which is also called the tocotransducer. When the pregnant woman feels the fetus move, she can make a mark on a graph paper that displays the fetal heart rate and the uterine activity. When the fetus moves, the fetal heart rate usually increases. It's just like the condition that a person's heart beats fast when he or she does exercise. Certain changes in the fetal heart rate are considered a sign of good health.

The treatment should depend on the levels of PIH. If PIH is mild, it can be treated at home. The mother needs to maintain a quiet and restful environment with limited activity or bed rest with doctor's advice. If PIH becomes worse, go to hospital immediately where both the pregnant woman and the baby can be closely monitored. In severe cases, both the mother and the baby are at the risk of dying. The baby has to be delivered.

🎧 Key Words

pre-eclampsia / ˌpriːɪˈklæmpsiə / n.
子痫前期，先兆子痫
fluid / ˈfluːɪd / n. 流体；液体
retention / rɪˈtenʃn / n. 滞留；闭尿
reflex / ˈriːfleks / n. 反射
dizziness / ˈdɪzinəs / n. 头晕；头昏眼花

kidney / ˈkɪdni / n. 肾脏
delivery / dɪˈlɪvəri / n. 分娩
diagnose / ˈdaɪəgnəʊz / v. 诊断；断定
prenatal / ˌpriːˈneɪtl / adj. 产前的；胎儿期的
uterine / ˈjuːtəraɪn / adj. 子宫的
tocotransducer / ˌtəʊkəʊtrænzˈdjuːsə(r) / n. 分娩换能器

Useful Expressions

pregnancy toxemia　妊娠毒血症
pregnancy-induced hypertension(PIH)
妊娠高血压综合征

pregnancy complication　妊娠并发症
systolic and diastolic pressures　收缩压和舒张压
ultrasound transducer　超声波传感器

Exercise

Ⅰ Choose the best answer to each question based on the text.

1. When does PIH occur? _____.

　A. After the 20th week of pregnancy

　B. Before the 20th week of pregnancy

　C. After being pregnant

2. What are the symptoms of PIH mentioned in the text? _____.

　A. Rapid or sudden weight loss, high blood pressure, and swelling (in the hands, feet, and face)

B. Rapid or sudden weight gain, hypertension, protein in the urine, and swelling (in the hands, feet, and face)

C. High blood pressure, protein in the blood, and swelling (in the hands, feet, and face)

3. Who is at the risk of having PIH? _____.

A. Women who are over 40

B. Women whose mothers and sisters had PIH

C. Both A and B

4. Which of the following statements is NOT true according to the text? _____.

A. No one test diagnoses PIH

B. If the fetal heart rate increases, it's the sign of danger

C. PIH can develop after delivery

5. When a pregnant woman gets PIH, she _____.

A. must go to hospital immediately

B. can be treated at home

C. has to give birth

II Match each medical term in Column A with its explanation in Column B.

Column A	Column B
_____ 1. pre-eclampsia	a. blood poisoning caused by bacterial toxic substances in the blood
_____ 2. tocotransducer	b. one of the symptoms of PIH
_____ 3. proteinuria	c. a pressure transducer
_____ 4. toxemia	d. protein in the urine
_____ 5. PIH	e. pregnancy-induced hypertension

III Find words or terms in the article to match the following definitions.

1. a pregnancy complication characterized by high blood pressure, swelling and protein in the urine _____

2. an abnormal accumulation of clear, watery fluid in the tissues or cavities of the body _____

3. the symptom of an abnormal enlargement of a body's part or area _____

4. the symptom of systolic and diastolic pressures equal to or exceed 140/90 mmHg _____

5. the process of giving birth to a baby _____

IV Critical thinking.

According to the case at the beginning of this unit, what are the nursing diagnoses and the nursing interventions for the patient?

1. Nursing diagnoses

• Altered tissue perfusion related to increased vascular resistance

• Fluid volume excess related to sodium and fluid retention

• Anxiety related to the fear of any influence on the baby

2. Nursing interventions

The patient and family members need information in order to know the name and the dosage of the drug, the frequency of taking the drug and the possible side effects. Adequate rest and sleep must be guaranteed. The nurse must instruct the patient to take the left lateral position to improve blood supply to the uterus and placenta. Maintaining adequate protein and calcium intake and restricting sodium intake in the daily diet. Moderate exercise should be encouraged as a way to control weight. Teaching about the hypertension and the potential complications to the patient and the family is essential to help relieve the anxiety.

Part 4 Supplementary Reading

🎧 Blue Light Therapy

Blue light therapy becomes photodynamic therapy when it uses the combination of photosynthesizing (or light-sensitive) drugs and a high-intensity light source to activate them. The light uses a natural violet or blue light, which can kill bad bacteria, help regulate mood and body clock as well as supporting the patient's livers. It can also deal with some health issues, such as acne, MRSA (methicillin-resistant staphylococcus aureus), depression, disorders, periodontal disease, neonatal jaundice, liver issues.

Blue light therapy also has a lot of advantages. It's 100% natural and drug free. It doesn't damage the skin without needles or knives, so it's painless. It's safe for all ages and all skin types, and it can even shine on the most delicate and tender newborn babies' skin, and there are no short- or long-term side effects. Therefore, it is also a favourite treatment for neonatal jaundice.

What is neonatal jaundice? It is a yellowish discoloration of the white part of the eyes and skin in a newborn baby due to high-level bilirubin in blood. It is estimated that three out of five infants have neonatal jaundice within the first month of life, so it is a common condition among newborn babies. Though some cases of neonatal jaundice will disappear on its own within a week or two, others require additional treatment.

The process of blue light phototherapy allows the blue light to be absorbed by the skin and the capillaries of the baby, enabling the body to change the bilirubin in the blood so that it can move through the system and be passed. During the process, the baby should be undressed but wear a diaper so that as much of the skin as possible is exposed to the light. The baby's eyes should be covered with a special soft eye protection to protect from the bright light. There is no need to stop breastfeeding, and feeding should continue on a regular time. The bilirubin level should be focused on and measured at least once a day. When the baby is not distressed, he or she will move less. Therefore, the processes of the blue light therapy are most effective due to the light that will better stay in the same place.

Blue light therapy will effectively lower the bilirubin to safe levels, so it's a very safe treatment method that has been used for years without reports of adverse side effects.

Exercise

Choose the best answer to each question based on the text.

1. Blue light therapy uses a combination of _____ or _____ to activate them.

    A. a natural violet light; a natural blue light

    B. light-sensitive drugs; a high-intensity light source

    C. light-sensitive drugs; photosynthesizing drugs

2. The following are the advantages of blue light therapy except it is _____.

    A. 100% natural and drug free

    B. painless

    C. very expensive

3. Which of the following statements is true according to the text? _____.

    A. Neonatal jaundice is a common condition among newborn babies

    B. Neonatal jaundice won't disappear if there's no additional treatment

    C. Blue light therapy is a favourite treatment for neonatal jaundice because it's very convenient

4. During the process of blue light therapy, the baby should be _____.

    A. undressed but wear a diaper

    B. covered with a special soft eye protection

    C. both A and B

5. How often should bilirubin level be measured a day? _____.

    A. At least once   B. No more than twice   C. As many times as possible

Part 5 Medical Word Elements

1. gynec(o)-   女性
    gynecology / ˌɡaɪnəˈkɒlədʒi /   遗传生态学
    gynecopathy / ˌɡaɪnɪˈkɒpəθi /   妇科病
2. uter(o)-   子宫
    uterotonic / ˌjuːtərəʊˈtɒnɪk /   子宫收缩剂
    uterotomy / ˌjuːtəˈrɒtəmi /   子宫切开术
3. mamm(o)-   乳房，乳腺
    mammogenesis / ˌmæməˈdʒenɪsɪs /   乳腺发育
    mammogram / ˈmæməɡræm /   乳房 X 线照片
4. men(o)-   月经
    menopausal / ˌmenəˈpɔːzl /   绝经期的
    menorrhagia / ˌmenəˈreɪdʒiə /   月经过多

5. ovari(o)-　　　　　　　　　　　　　　　　　卵巢
   ovariocyesis / əʊˌveəriəʊsaɪˈiːsɪs /　　　卵巢妊娠
   ovariorrhexis / əʊˌveəriəʊˈrekəsɪs /　　卵巢破裂
6. cervic(o)-　　　　　　　　　　　　　　　　　子宫颈
   cervicoplasty / ˈsəːvikəuˌplæsti /　　　宫颈成形术
   cervicovaginal / ˌsɜːvɪkəʊˈvædʒɪnl /　　子宫颈阴道的
7. vagin(o)-　　　　　　　　　　　　　　　　　阴道
   vaginocele / ˈvædʒɪnəsiːl /　　　　　　阴道脱垂
   vaginoplasty / vəˈdʒaɪnəʊˌplæsti /　　阴道成形术
8. ureter(o)-　　　　　　　　　　　　　　　　　输尿管
   ureterolith / jʊəˈriːtərəlɪθ /　　　　　输尿管石
   ureteropyosis / jʊəˌriːtərəʊpaɪˈəʊsɪs /　输尿管化脓
9. urethr(o)-　　　　　　　　　　　　　　　　　尿道
   urethrism / jʊəˈriːθrɪzəm /　　　　　　尿道痉挛
   urethrostaxis / jʊəˌriːθrəʊˈstæksɪs /　尿道渗血

（韩亚蕾　赵　静）

Caring for a Patient with Stroke

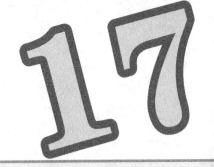

Learning Objectives:

1. *Discussing the effects of stroke*
2. *Describing the procedures of performing defibrillation*
3. *Defining cerebrovascular accidents (CVAs), their symptoms and therapies*
4. *Understanding and explaining neurosurgery*

Lead-In

Case Study

Michael Jackson was a 70-year-old retired worker who was brought to the emergency department by his wife. She noticed that all of sudden her husband "was slurring his speech and his face was drooping on one side". Michael Jackson told his wife that he felt some numbness on the right side of his face and in his right arm. Michael Jackson's wife was afraid her husband was having a stroke so she brought him to hospital. Michael Jackson did not have a headache and denied any nausea, vomiting, chest pain, diaphoresis, or visual complaints.

Part 1 Dialogue

🎧 Discussing the Effects of Stroke

Michael Jackson, a 70-year-old retired worker, has just suffered from a stroke. Elizabeth, the ward nurse, talks to his daughter, Helen Jackson, about the structure of brain and what happens in the ischaemic stroke.

Elizabeth: Right. Let's look at the structure of the brain first. The brain is divided into two hemispheres, or parts. The Circle of Willis allows blood to branch out and reach the entire brain. The left and right carotid arteries supply oxygenated blood to the brain.

Helen: Of course, "hemi" means half, doesn't it?

Elizabeth: That's right. Ischaemia results from a blockage in a cerebral blood vessel and causes the brain to be deprived of oxygen and important nutrients. Thrombi which lodge in any of the blood vessels of the brain may obstruct the blood flow. The formation of a blood clot in a patient's brain or in one of his/her blood vessels makes thrombosis, which can cause stroke.

Helen:	My father suffered a stroke, right?
Elizabeth:	Yes, that's right. Ischaemic stroke is the most common stroke, which accounts for 80% of all the strokes. Haemorrhagic stroke is less common, and accounts for 20% of all the strokes. Both can cause death.
Helen:	Fortunately, we sent him to hospital in time.
Elizabeth:	Yeah, but some complications occurred, such as right hemiplegia, or right-sided paralysis, dysphagia, or dysphagia, dysarthria, or difficulty articulating words, and he needs a long time to recover.
Helen:	My father seems to have problems finding the right words, too.
Elizabeth:	Some patients also have aphasia, or an inability to communicate. Fortunately, your father is able to communicate, but he does have dysphasia, or difficulty expressing himself. That's why he says the wrong words for the thought he's trying to express.
Helen:	It's a real problem. It's really frustrating him. We don't know what to do.
Elizabeth:	Mm, emotional lability is very common. It usually shows up as crying at inappropriate time, but it can also be laughing or giggling. It's very distressing, I know.
Helen:	Oh, OK. Thanks for explaining that. We'll try to be more patient with him. He's also so slow at the moment. Why's that?
Elizabeth:	People who have had a stroke tend to have a slow and cautious behaviour pattern. You'll need to repeat any instruction you give to your father a few times before he'll understand them. Besides, he has memory loss: his short-term memory has been affected.
Helen:	Yes, I've noticed that. Thank you for your patient explanations.
Elizabeth:	Oh, I'm glad to do that.

🎧 Key Words

hemisphere / 'hemisfiə(r) / n. 半球
ischaemia / ɪ'skiːmiə / n. 局部缺血
cerebral / 'serəbrəl / adj. 脑的
thrombosis / θrɒm'bəʊsɪs / n. 血栓形成
haemorrhagic / hemə'rædʒɪk / adj. 出血的
hemiplegia / ˌhemɪ'pliːdʒiə / n. 偏瘫

paralysis / pə'ræləsɪs / n. 麻痹；瘫痪
dysphagia / dɪs'feɪdʒiə / n. 咽下困难
dysarthria / dɪs'ɑːθriə / n. 构音困难
articulate / ɑː'tɪkjuleɪt / v. 清晰地发（音）
aphasia / ə'feɪziə / n. 失语症
lability / lə'bɪləti / n. 易变性

Useful Expressions

ischaemic stroke　缺氧性脑中风
Circle of Willis　动脉环，韦利斯环
carotid arteries　颈动脉

blood vessel　血管
short-term memory　短时记忆

Exercise

Ⅰ **Read the dialogue again and decide whether the following statements are right or wrong. If there is not enough information to answer "Right" or "Wrong", choose "Doesn't say".**

1. The brain is divided into two hemispheres, and the Circle of Willis allows blood to branch out and reach the entire brain._____.

   A. Right   B. Wrong   C. Doesn't say

2. The haemorrhagic stroke is the most common stroke which accounts for 80% of all the strokes. _____.

   A. Right   B. Wrong   C. Doesn't say

3. Helen's father seems to have no problems finding the right words. _____.

   A. Right   B. Wrong   C. Doesn't say

4. People who have had a stroke tend to have a slow and cautious behaviour pattern._____.

   A. Right   B. Wrong   C. Doesn't say

5. It is important to be patient when you talk to someone who has had a stroke because he/she can't hear properly. _____.

   A. Right   B. Wrong   C. Doesn't say

Ⅱ **Discussion.**

What symptoms do people who have had a stroke have and what should their families pay special attention to?

Part 2 Short Passage

🎧 Performing Defibrillation

An automated external defibrillator (AED) is an electronic device that automatically diagnoses the life-threatening cardiac arrhythmias of ventricular fibrillation and pulseless ventricular tachycardia, and is able to treat them through defibrillation, the application of electricity which stops the arrhythmia, allowing the heart to reestablish an effective rhythm. With simple audio and visual commands, AEDs are simple to use for the layperson, and the use of AEDs is taught in first aid, certified first responders, and cardiopulmonary resuscitation (CPR) classes at basic life support (BLS) level.

When turned on or opened, the AED will instruct the user to connect the electrodes (pads) to the patient. Once the pads are attached, everyone should avoid touching the patient so as to avoid false readings by the unit. The pads allow the AED to examine the electrical output from the heart and determine if the patient is in a shockable rhythm (either ventricular fibrillation or ventricular tachycardia). If the device determines that a shock is warranted, it will use the battery to charge its internal capacitor in preparation for the shock. This system is not only safer (charging only when required), but also allows a faster delivery of the electric currents. When charged, the device instructs the user to ensure no one is touching the patient and then to press a button to deliver the shock;

human intervention is usually required to deliver the shock to the patient in order to avoid the possibility of accidental injury to another person (which can result from a responder or bystander touching the patient at the time of the shock). Depending on the manufacturer and the particular model, after the shock is delivered most devices will analyze the patient and either instruct CPR to be performed, or prepare to administer another shock.

The following procedures will show how to perform defibrillation in hospitals.

1. Place the paddles on the saline pads. Ensure that the defibrillator is charged to 350 to 400 watt seconds.

2. Instruct all persons to move away from the bed area.

3. Press the discharge buttons on the defibrillator simultaneously to ensure appropriate energy discharge.

4. Check the ECG pattern to determine the effects of the defibrillation. Reinstitute CPR and administer sodium bicarbonate or other appropriate medications if the ventricular fibrillation continues.

5. Prepare the defibrillator equipment for the second attempt.

6. Instruct all the persons to move away from the bed area.

7. Repeat the defibrillation procedure.

8. Monitor the patient every 15 minutes after defibrillation until the condition is stable .

9. Continue the oxygen administration.

10. Continue the IV medication administration, e.g., antiarrhythmics, vasopressors, etc.

11. Monitor the ECG strips continuously until the condition is stable.

12. Observe for the ECG signs of the pacemaker malfunction.

13. Maintain patient on bed rest.

🎧 Key Words

defibrillation / ˌdiːfɪbrɪˈleɪʃn / n. 除颤
defibrillator / diːˈfɪbrɪleɪtə(r) / n. 除颤器
ventricular / venˈtrɪkjələ(r) / adj. 心室的
fibrillation / ˌfaɪbrɪˈleɪʃn / n. 纤维性颤动
electrode / ɪˈlektrəʊd / n. 电极

capacitor / kəˈpæsɪtə(r) / n. 电容器
antiarrhythmic / ˌænʃiəˈrɪðmɪk / n. 抗心律失常药
vasopressor / veɪzəʊˈpresə(r) / n. 血管加压药
malfunction / mælˈfʌŋkʃn / n. 功能障碍

Useful Expressions

automated external defibrillator (AED)　自动
体外除颤器
ventricular fibrillation　心室颤动

pulseless ventricular tachycardia　无脉搏的室
性心动过速
basic life support (BLS)　基础生命支持
sodium bicarbonate　碳酸氢钠

Exercise

▌ Choose the best answer to each question based on the text.

1. An automated external defibrillator (AED) is an electronic device that automatically diagnoses the

life-threatening _____, and both can be treated through defibrillation.

A. cardiac arrhythmias of ventricular fibrillation and pulseless ventricular tachycardia

B. cardiac arrest and bradycardia

C. cardiac failure and myocardial infarction

2. Once the pads of AEDs are attached, _____ should avoid touching the patient so as to avoid false readings by the unit.

    A. no one   B. someone   C. everyone

3. Human intervention is _____ required to deliver the shock to the patient in order to avoid the possibility of accidental injury to another person.

    A. usually   B. never   C. seldom

4. When using defibrillator, one should first place paddles on the saline pads and ensure that the defibrillator is charged to _____ seconds.

    A. 350 to 400 watt   B. 200 to 250 watt   C. 250 to 300 watt

5. After the defibrillation is performed, the patient should be monitored every _____ until the condition is stable.

    A. 10 minutes   B. 15 minutes   C. 20 minutes

II **Read the passage again and put the following extracts in the correct order.**

☐ **A** Instruct all the persons to move away from the bed area.

☐ **B** Check the ECG pattern to determine the effects of the defibrillation, and administer oxygen and some appropriate medications if the ventricular fibrillation continues.

☐ **C** Press the discharge buttons on the defibrillator meanwhile to ensure appropriate energy discharge.

☐ **D** Maintain the patient the on bed rest.

☐ **E** Monitor ECG strips continuously until the condition is stable and observe for the ECG signs of pacemaker malfunction.

☐ **F** Place the paddles on the saline pads and ensure that the defibrillator is charged to 350 to 400 watt seconds.

☐ **G** Monitor the patient every 15 minutes after defibrillation until the condition is stable.

Part 3 Text

🎧 Cerebrovascular Accidents (CVA)

Cerebrovascular accidents (CVA) include the disorders that cause interruptions in the blood supply to or within the brain. Examples of these are embolism, thrombosis, ruptured cerebral aneurysms, and intracerebral and subarachnoid hemorrhages. The most common presentation of cerebrovascular accidents is an ischaemic stroke and sometimes a hemorrhagic stroke.

The most common cerebrovascular diseases is an acute stroke, which occurs when blood supply to the brain is compromised. Symptoms of a stroke are usually rapid at the onset, and may in clude hemiparesis, hemiplegia, dysphasia, dysphagia and dysarthria. Hemorrhagic strokes can present a very severe, sudden headache associated with vomiting, neck stiffness, vision changes, balance difficulties, and decreased consciousness. Symptoms vary depending on the location and the size of the area involved in the stroke. Edema, or swelling of the brain may increase the intracranial pressure and result in brain herniation. A stroke may result in coma or death if it involves the key areas of the brain.

Other symptoms of the cerebrovascular accidents include migraines, seizures, epilepsy, or cognitive decline. However, cerebrovascular diseases may go undetected for years until an acute stroke occurs. In addition, patients with some rare congenital cerebrovascular diseases may begin to have these symptoms in childhood.

Control of hypertension (the major risk factor for all the types of stroke), can decrease the incidence of stroke. Other major risk factors for stroke include advancing age, a history of a transient ischaemic attack, reversible ischaemic neurologic deficit, prior stroke, diabetes and atrial fibrillation. There are also many less common causes of cerebrovascular disease, including those that are congenital or idiopathic and also including CADASIL, aneurysms, amyloid angiopathy, arteriovenous malformations, fistulas, and arterial dissections. Many of these diseases can be asymptomatic until an acute event, such as a stroke, occurs. Cerebrovascular diseases can also present themselves less commonly with headaches or seizures. Any of these diseases can result in vascular dementia due to ischaemic damage to the brain.

The acquired cerebrovascular accidents may be obtained throughout a person's life and may be preventable by controlling the risk factors. The incidence of cerebrovascular disease increases as an individual ages. Causes of the acquired cerebrovascular disease include arteriosclerosis, embolism, aneurysms, and arterial dissections. Arteriosclerosis leads to the narrowing of the blood vessels and less perfusion to the brain, and it also increases the risk of thrombosis, or a blockage of an artery, within the brain. The major modifiable risk factors for arteriosclerosis include: hypertension, smoking, obesity and diabetes.

Treatment for cerebrovascular accidents may include medication, lifestyle changes and/or surgery, depending on the causes.

Emergency measures of the CVAs victims include the following.

1. Turn the patient onto the affected side.

2. Elevate the head without flexing the neck.

3. Loose the tight clothing.

4. Keep the patient warm and quiet.

5. Comfort the patient.

6. Ask for medical help.

🎧 Key Words

aneurysm / ˈænjəˌrɪzəm / n. 动脉瘤   subarachnoid / ˌsʌbəˈræknɔɪd, / adj. 蛛网膜下腔的

compromise / ˈkɒmprəmaɪz / v. 妥协，折中；使陷入危险

dysphasia / dɪsˈfeɪziə / n. 言语困难症

intracranial / ˌɪntrəˈkreɪniəl / adj. 颅内的

migraine / ˈmaɪgreɪn / n. 偏头痛

seizure / ˈsiːʒə(r) / n. 惊厥

epilepsy / ˈepɪlepsi / n. 癫痫

idiopathic / ˌɪdɪəˈpæθɪk / adj. 先天的

amyloid / ˈæmɪlɔɪd / adj. 淀粉样的

fistula / ˈfɪstjʊlə / n. 瘘管

asymptomatic / əˌsɪmptəˈmætɪk / adj. 无症状的

dementia / dɪˈmenʃə / n. 痴呆

arteriosclerosis / ɑːˌtɪəriəʊskləˈrəʊsɪs / n. 动脉硬化

Useful Expressions

subarachnoid hemorrhage　蛛网膜下腔出血
brain herniation　脑疝
cognitive decline　认知减退
congenital cerebrovascular disease　先天性脑血管疾病
transient ischemic attack　短暂性脑缺血发作

atrial fibrillation　房颤
amyloid angiopathy　淀粉样血管病变
arteriovenous malformation　动静脉畸形
arterial dissection　动脉剥离

Exercise

Ⅰ Choose the best answer to each question based on the text.

1. Cerebrovascular accidents (CVA) include the disorders that cause interruptions in the blood supply _____.

   A. to or within the lungs

   B. to or within the heart

   C. to or within the brain

2. The most common presentation of cerebrovascular accidents is _____.

   A. an ischaemic stroke

   B. sometimes a hemorrhagic stroke

   C. both A and B

3. Symptoms vary depending on _____ of the area involved in the stroke.

   A. the location and the size

   B. the type

   C. the blockage level

4. Treatment for cerebrovascular accidents may include _____ depending on the cause.

   A. a balanced diet and physical exercise

   B. medication, lifestyle changes and/or surgery

   C. quitting smoking and eating food rich in protein

5. Emergency measures of the CVAs victim include the following except _____.

   A. turning the patient onto the affected side and elevating the head without flexing the neck

   B. loosening tight clothing and keeping the patient warm and quiet

   C. giving the patient CPR and administering oxygen therapy

II **Match each medical term in Column A with its explanation in Column B.**

	Column A	Column B
_____	1. intracranial	a. a medical condition in which one's arteries become hard and thick
_____	2. arteriosclerosis	b. paralysis of one side of the body
_____	3. hemiplegia	c. within the skull
_____	4. dysphagia	d. mental deterioration of organic or functional origin
_____	5. dementia	e. a condition in which swallowing is difficult or painful

III **Find words or terms in the article to match the following definitions.**

1. impaired articulatory ability resulting from defects in the peripheral motor nerves or in the speech musculature _____

2. present at birth but not necessarily hereditary _____

3. the formation of a blood clot in the heart or in one of the blood vessels, which can cause death _____

4. swelling from excessive accumulation of serous fluid in tissue _____

IV **Critical thinking.**

According to the case at the beginning of this unit, what are nursing diagnoses and nursing interventions for the patient?

1. Nursing diagnoses

- Altered physical mobility related to hemiparesis
- Risk for injury related to impaired mobility
- Impaired verbal communication related to dysarthria

2. Nursing interventions

Maintaining blood pressure and providing hydration are important interventions at this time. Early mobilization of the patients with stroke is beneficial for long-term functional outcome. Maintaining a normal bowel and bladder elimination are also important nursing goals. It's important to encourage the patient to use verbal communication and provide a comfortable and caring environment. The nurse should support and protect the patient from injury.

Part 4 Supplementary Reading

🎧 Neurosurgery

Neurosurgery is the medical speciality concerned with the prevention, diagnosis, surgical treatment, and rehabilitation of disorders which affect the nervous system including the brain, spinal cord, peripheral nerves, and cerebrovascular system.

Neuroradiology methods are used in modern neurosurgery diagnosis and treatment. They include computer-assisted imaging computerized tomography (CT), magnetic resonance imaging (MRI), positron emission tomography (PET), magnetoencephalography (MEG), and stereotactic radiosurgery. Some neurosurgery procedures involve the use of intra-operative MRI and functional MRI.

In conventional open surgery the neurosurgeon opens the skull, creating a large opening to access the brain. Techniques involving smaller openings with the aid of microscopes and endoscopes are now being used as well. Methods that utilize small craniotomies in conjunction with high-clarity microscopic visualization of neural tissue offer excellent results. However, the open methods are still traditionally used in trauma or emergency situations.

Microsurgery is utilized in many aspects of neurological surgery. Microvascular techniques are used in IC EC bypass surgery and in restoration carotid endarterectomy. The clipping of an aneurysm is performed under microscopic vision. Minimally invasive spine surgery utilizes microscopes or endoscopes. Procedures such as microdiscectomy, laminectomy, and artificial disc replacement rely on microsurgery.

Using stereotaxy neurosurgeons can approach a minute target in the brain through a minimal opening. This is used in functional neurosurgery where electrodes are implanted or gene therapy is instituted with a high level of accuracy as in the case of Parkinson's disease or Alzheimer's disease. Using the combination method of open and stereotactic surgery, intraventricular hemorrhages can be potentially evacuated successfully. Conventional surgery using image guidance technologies is also becoming common and is referred to as surgical navigation, computer-assisted surgery, navigated surgery, and stereotactic navigation. Image-guided surgery systems, like curve image guided surgery and stealth station, use cameras or electromagnetic fields to capture and relay the patient's anatomy, and the surgeon's precise movements in relation to the patient, and to computer monitors in the operating room. These sophisticated computerized systems are used before and during the surgery to help orient the surgeon with three-dimensional images of the patient's anatomy including the tumour.

Minimally invasive endoscopic surgery is commonly utilized by neurosurgeons. Techniques such as endoscopic endonasal surgery are used in pituitary tumours, craniopharyngiomas, chordomas, and the repair of cerebrospinal fluid leaks. Ventricular endoscopy is used in the treatment of intraventricular bleeds, hydrocephalus, colloid cyst and neurocysticercosis. Endonasal endoscopy is at times carried out with neurosurgeons and ENT surgeons working together as a team.

Exercise

Choose the best answer to each question based on the text.

1. Neurosurgery is the medical speciality concerned with the disorders which affects _____.

    A. the nervous system

    B. the endocrine system

    C. the circulatory system

2. _____ are used in modern neurosurgery diagnosis and treatment.

    A. Neuroradiology methods

    B. Ultrasonic methods

C. Angiography methods

3. Using the combination method of open and stereotactic surgery, _____ can potentially be evacuated successfully.

  A. cerebral hemorrhages

  B. intraventricular hemorrhages

  C. gastric hemorrhages

4. _____ is used in the treatment of intraventricular bleeds, hydrocephalus, colloid cyst and neurocysticercosis.

  A. Endonasal endoscopy

  B. Ventricular microscopy

  C. Ventricular endoscopy

5. Techniques involving smaller openings with the aid of _____ are now being used widely.

  A. gastroscopes and nasoscopes

  B. arthroscopes and bronchoscopes

  C. microscopes and endoscopes

Part 5 Medical Word Elements

1. cephal(o)-   头

  cephalodynia / ˌsefələʊ'dɪnɪə /   头痛

  cephalotomy / ˌsefə'lɒtəmɪ /   穿颅术

2. cerebr(o)-   大脑

  cerebroma / ˌserɪ'brəʊmə /   脑瘤

  cerebrum / se'riːbrəm /   大脑

3. encephal(o)-   脑

  encephalalgia / enˌsefə'lældʒɪə /   头痛

  encephalorrhagia / enˌsefələʊ'reɪdʒɪə /   脑出血

4. cerebell(o)-   小脑

  cerebellum / ˌserɪ'beləm /   小脑

  cerebellospinal / ˌserɪˌbeləʊ'spaɪnl /   小脑脊髓的

5. crani(o)-   颅

  craniopuncture / 'kreɪnɪəˌpʌŋktʃər /   颅穿刺术

  craniology / ˌkreɪnɪ'ɒlədʒi /   颅骨学

6. neur(o)-   神经

  neuroanatomy / ˌnjʊərəʊə'nætəmi /   神经解剖学

  neuroglia / njʊə'rɒglɪə /   神经胶质

7. gangli(o)-   神经节

  gangliocytoma / ˌgæŋglɪəʊsaɪ'təʊmə /   神经节细胞瘤

ganglioneuroma /ˌɡæŋɡlɪəʊnjʊəˈrəʊmə /	神经节细胞瘤
8. scler(o)-	硬化
scleredema /ˌsklɪərɪˈdiːmə /	硬肿症
scleroderma /ˌsklɪərəʊˈdɜːmə /	硬皮病
9. mening(o)-	脑膜，脑脊膜
meningitis /ˌmenɪnˈdʒaɪtɪs /	脑膜炎
meningoencephalitis /məˌnɪŋɡəʊenˌsefəˈlaɪtɪs /	脑膜脑炎

（王炎峰　赵　静）

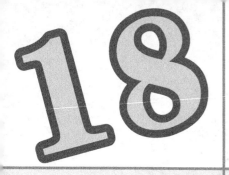

Caring for a Patient with Alzheimer's Disease

Learning Objectives:

1. *Educating a relative of the patient with Alzheimer's disease*
2. *Discussing the four stages of Alzheimer's disease*
3. *Describing the nursing interventions in Alzheimer's disease*
4. *Providing information about the relaxation therapy*

Lead-In

Case Study

A 79-year-old American lady lived independently at home; she fell and sustained a hip fracture. Medical history revealed only hypertension. Her family noted she was "very different" from before. They admitted she had been getting a "little forgetful". Discharged to home, it soon became apparent that she couldn't perform the activities of daily living, and she was transferred to a health care facility. After a series of tests including a lumbar puncture for cerebrospinal fluid (CSF) biomarkers, she was diagnosed with Alzheimer's dementia by a geriatric neurologist.

Part 1 Dialogue

🎧 Educating a Relative of the Patient with Alzheimer's Disease

Mr. Clausen, whose mother is a patient with Alzheimer's disease, is complaining of something wrong with his mother. Alexandra, the ward nurse, is listening and educating him about the symptoms and interventions for Alzheimer's disease.

Mr. Clausen: I can't take this another day. Now I am being accused of stealing my mother's underwear.

Alexandra: Oh, I understand. Your mother suffers from Alzheimer's disease(AD). This must be a difficult time for you and your mother.

Mr. Clausen: Alzheimer's disease? That is dementia?

Alexandra:	Yes, also called dementia of the Alzheimer type, it is a chronic disease. A patient who has Alzheimer's disease will struggle in it three to ten years.
Mr. Clausen:	Ten years? Is it curable?
Alexandra:	No, it is incurable. Some famous persons, for example, Mrs. Margaret Hilda Thatcher and Ronald Wilson Reagan, died of this disease. I'm sorry to tell you this.
Mr. Clausen:	Oh, my poor mother! What can I do for her?
Alexandra:	Your mother has long-term memory loss and disorientation, which are the symptoms at the middle stage of AD. Dr. Vitellius will prescribe some Donepezil which can improve her memory.
Mr. Clausen:	Oh, I'll let her take medicine in time. What else could I do?
Alexandra:	Talk more about something happy in the past with her, and promote independence in her self-care as much as possible.
Mr. Clausen:	Promote independence? What do you mean?
Alexandra:	Independence in self-care can give her a sense of achievement. So let her do self-care as much as possible. For example, when you tell her to brush her teeth, it may be necessary to give her step-by-step directions.
Mr. Clausen:	What can we do for her memory loss?
Alexandra:	Establish a routine schedule of activities for her. Call her name, tell her where she is, and state your name at each contact with her. On the wall, hang up an electric clock with the date and o'clock alarm.
Mr. Clausen:	She always loses her way, even at home. How to manage?
Alexandra:	When she goes for a walk, you or other persons must accompany her. She needs a bracelet or a necklace with your contact number in case of her wandering. Write signs on the door, especially the washroom.
Mr. Clausen:	What is the best place that my mother can live in now?
Alexandra:	Of course, at home. Make home as safe and familiar as possible. Don't change the furnishings in the house, especially in your mother's room. But if you think your mother is out of control and you can't take it anymore someday, we should explore alternative care settings for her.

🎧 Key Words

curable / ˈkjʊərəbl / *adj.* 可治愈的
disorientation / dɪsˌɔːriənˈteɪʃn / *n.* 定向障碍
Donepezil / dəˈnɪpəzɪl / *n.* 多奈哌齐
independence / ˌɪndɪˈpendəns / *n.* 独立性，自立性
achievement / əˈtʃiːvmənt / *n.* 成就

bracelet / ˈbreɪslət / *n.* 手镯
necklace / ˈnekləs / *n.* 项链
wandering / ˈwɒndərɪŋ / *n.* 漫游；流浪
furnishing / ˈfɜːnɪʃɪŋ / *n.* 家具陈设
alternative / ɔːlˈtɜːnətɪv / *adj.* 供替代的

Useful Expressions

Alzheimer's disease(AD) 阿尔茨海默症，
老年痴呆症
step-by-step direction 一步一步的指导

memory loss 记忆丧失
routine schedule of activities 日常活动时间表
care settings 医疗设置

Exercise

I **Read the dialogue again and decide whether the following statements are right or wrong. If there is not enough information to answer "Right" or "Wrong", choose "Doesn't say".**

1. Alzheimer's disease, also called dementia of the Alzheimer type, is an acute disease. _____.

   A. Right   B. Wrong   C. Doesn't say

2. Short-term memory loss is the symptoms at the middle stage of AD. _____.

   A. Right   B. Wrong   C. Doesn't say

3. Some medications can improve AD patients' memory. _____.

   A. Right   B. Wrong   C. Doesn't say

4. Promoting AD patients' independence in self-care as much as possible is crucial. _____.

   A. Right   B. Wrong   C. Doesn't say

5. The place where AD patients live should be as safe and familiar as possible. _____.

   A. Right   B. Wrong   C. Doesn't say

II **Discussion.**

What information might you need to talk about when educating a relative of the patient with Alzheimer's disease?

Part 2 Short Passage

🎧 Stages of Alzheimer's Disease

Alzheimer's disease (AD) is a chronic neurodegenerative disease that usually starts slowly and worsens over time. The disease course is divided into four stages, with a progressive pattern of cognitive and functional impairment.

Stage 1: Mild Alzheimer's Disease

The most noticeable deficit is short-term memory loss, or forgetfulness. The person with mild AD loses energy, drive, and initiative and has difficulty learning new things, but personality and social behaviour remain intact. The individual may still continue to work, but the extent of the dementia becomes evident in a new or demanding situation. Depression may occur early in the disease but usually lessens as the disease progresses. Activities such as doing the marketing or managing finances are noticeably impaired during this phase.

Stage 2: Moderate Alzheimer's Disease

The person with moderate AD can't remember his or her address or date. Hygiene suffers and the person has to be coaxed to bathe. The ability to dress appropriately is markedly affected. Often, the mood becomes labile, and the individual may have bursts of paranoia, anger, jealousy, and apathy. Activities such as driving become hazardous. Care and supervision become a full-time job for family members. Denial mercifully takes over and protects people from the realization that they are losing control. People begin to withdraw from activities and others. The person may also have moments of becoming tearful and sad.

Stage 3: Moderate to Severe Alzheimer's Disease

At this stage, the person is often unable to identify familiar objects or people, even a spouse. The person needs repeated instructions and directions for the simplest tasks, such as washing face. Often, the individual can't remember where the toilet is and becomes incontinent. Total care is necessary and the burden on the family can be emotionally, financially, and physically devastating. Agitation, violence, paranoia, and delusions are commonly seen. Another problem, wandering behaviour, can make the person at the risk of becoming lost. Institutionalization may be the most appropriate recourse at this time.

Stage 4: Late Stage Alzheimer's Disease

The person loses the ability to read and write and to recognize familiar objects. He has the need to taste, chew, and put everything in his mouth, and to touch everything in sight. At this stage, the abilities to talk and walk are lost eventually. Seizures and primitive reflexes may develop. If death due to secondary causes, such as infection or choking, has not come, the end stage of AD is characterized by stupor and coma.

🎧 Key Words

neurodegenerative / ˌnjuːrəʊdɪˈdʒenərətɪv / adj. 神经变性的

progressive / prəˈgresɪv / adj. 越来越严重的

cognitive / ˈkɒgnətɪv / adj. 认知的

deficit / ˈdefɪsɪt / n. 不足

personality / ˌpɜːsəˈnæləti / n. 个性；性格

depression / dɪˈpreʃn / n. 抑郁，抑郁症

coax / kəʊks / v. 哄，劝诱；哄骗

paranoia / ˌpærəˈnɔɪə / n. 妄想症；偏执狂

hazardous / ˈhæzədəs / adj. 冒险的，有危险的

mercifully / ˈmɜːsɪfəli / adv. 仁慈地

devastating / ˈdevəsteɪtɪŋ / adj. 毁灭性的

delusion / dɪˈluːʒn / n. 妄想

institutionalization / ˌɪnstɪˌtjuːʃənəlaɪˈzeɪʃn / n. 收容在专门机构（精神病院、教养所）

recourse / rɪˈkɔːs / n. 求助；求援的对象

stupor / ˈstjuːpə(r) / n.（精神）恍惚

Useful Expressions

chronic neurodegenerative disease	慢性神经退行性疾病	social behaviour	社会性行为
cognitive and functional impairment	认知和功能障碍	primitive reflex	原始反射

Exercise

I Choose the best answer to each question based on the text.

1. Alzheimer's disease (AD) is a _____ disease with _____ impairment.

    A. chronic neurodegenerative; cognitive and behavioural

    B. acute neurodegenerative; affective disorder and functional

    C. chronic neurodegenerative; cognitive and functional

2. What are the symptoms of mild AD? _____.

    A. Short-term memory loss, intact personality and social behaviour

    B. Long-term memory loss, impaired personality and social behaviour

    C. Short-term memory loss, impaired personality and social behaviour

3. The individual with _____ may still continue to work.

    A. severe Alzheimer's disease

    B. moderate Alzheimer's disease

    C. mild Alzheimer's disease

4. _____ behaviour can make the person at the stage 3 of AD at the risk of being lost.

    A. Agitating   B. Wandering   C. Violent

5. At the late stage of Alzheimer's disease, _____ may develop.

    A. inability of identifying familiar objects or people

    B. ability to talk and walk

    C. seizures and primitive reflexes

II Read the passage again and put the following extracts in the correct order.

☐ **A** losing the abilities to talk and walk, being in stupor and coma

☐ **B** short-term memory loss and impaired ability to do things such as marketing or managing finances

☐ **C** bursts of paranoia, anger, jealousy, apathy and affected ability to dress appropriately

☐ **D** needs of repeated instructions and directions, incontinent

Part 3 Text

🎧 Alzheimer's Disease

Alzheimer's disease (AD) is commonly characterized by progressive deterioration of cognitive functioning. Initially deterioration may be so subtle and insidious that others may not notice. In the early stages of the disease, the affected person may be able to compensate for the loss of memory. Some people may have superior social grace and charm that give them the ability to hide severe deficits (denial) in the memory, even from the experienced health care professionals. As times goes, denial, confabulation, perseveration and avoidance of questions are four defensive behaviours for the client to maintain self-esteem. Cardinal symptoms observed in AD are aphasia (loss of the language ability), apraxia (loss of the purposeful movement in the absence of motor or sensory impairment), agnosia (loss of the sensory ability to recognize objects), memory impairment and disturbances in executive functioning (planning, organizing, abstract thinking).

Caring for a client with AD requires a great deal of patience, creativity, and maturity. The needs of such a client can be enormous for the nursing staff and for families who care for their loved ones in the home. The problems that may affect dementia sufferers and their families are memory impairment, disorientation, needs of physical help, risks in the home, risks outside, apathy, poor communication, repetitiveness, uncontrolled emotion, uncontrolled behaviour, incontinence, emotional reactions, mistaken beliefs, decision-making and a burden on family. Therefore, risk for injury, impaired verbal communication, impaired environmental interpretation syndrome and confusion occur. Ineffective coping, caregiver role strain and anticipatory grieving are also important phenomenon.

The basic principle underlying all the care for the cognitively impaired is to facilitate the highest level of functioning a person is capable in all area, e.g., self-care, social and family relationship. Communication guidelines for clients with AD include identifying the caregiver and calling the person by name at each meeting, using short, simple words and phrases, maintaining face-to-face contact, focusing on one piece of information at a time, talking with the client about familiar and meaningful things, and encouraging reminiscing about the happy time in life.

Family and health care guidelines for self-care are always having the client perform all the tasks within the capacity of the client's present condition, and giving step-by-step instruction whenever necessary. If the client is resistant to doing self-care, come back later and ask again. Monitor food and fluid intake, begin bowel and bladder program early. Maintain a calm atmosphere during the day, avoid the use of restraints, and give neuroleptics or sedative if necessary.

Have the client wear Medic-Alert bracelet with name, address, and telephone number that can't be removed. Encourage the client to do physical activities during the day. Label bathroom door as well as the doors to the other rooms. Have clocks, calendars, and family pictures in clear view of client to anchor client in reality.

The overall goals of the treatment are to promote the client's optimal level of functioning and to retard further regression, whenever possible. Working closely with the family and providing them with the names of available resources and support, may help improve the quality of life for both the family and the client.

🎧 Key Words

denial / dɪ'naɪəl / n. 否认
confabulation / kənˌfæbjə'leɪʃn / n. 虚构，虚构症
perseveration / pɜːˌsevə'reɪʃn / n. 持续言语，
持续重复的行为

apraxia / ei'præksiə / n. 失用，运用不能
agnosia / æg'nəʊziə / n. 失认，辨识不能
executive / ɪg'zekjətɪv / adj. 执行的，实施的
repetitiveness / rɪ'petətɪvnəs / n. 重复

reminisce / ˌremɪ'nɪs / vi. 追忆往事；怀旧
restraint / rɪ'streɪnt / n. 约束；限制
neuroleptic / ˌnjʊərəʊ'leptɪk / n. 安定药，
精神抑制药

sedative / 'sedətɪv / n. 镇静剂
anchor / 'æŋkə(r) / v. 固定，（使）稳定
retard / rɪ'tɑːd / v. 延迟，推迟
regression / rɪ'greʃn / n. 退化

Useful Expressions

social grace　社交风度，社交分寸
abstract thinking　抽象思维
risk for injury　有受伤的危险
impaired verbal communication　语言沟通障碍

impaired environmental interpretation syndrome
环境认知障碍综合征
role strain　角色压力，角色偏差
anticipatory grieving　预感性悲哀

Exercise

I Choose the best answer to each question based on the text.

1. In the early stages of AD, the affected person may _____.

A. not be able to compensate for the loss of memory

B. have the ability to hide severe deficits in the memory

C. not have disturbances in planning, organizing and abstract thinking

2. In the first paragraph, the word "confabulation" means _____.

A. an informal conversation

B. the act of persisting or persevering

C. a plausible but imagined memory that fills in gaps in what is remembered

3. Which of the following statements is true according to the text?_____.

A. A great deal of patience is required to care for a client with AD

B. The needs of a client with AD can be minimal

C. Memory impairment and disorientation won't occur for a client with AD

4. Communication guidelines for clients with AD include the following except _____.

A. calling the person by name at each meeting

B. using short, simple words and phrases

C. encouraging reminiscing about difficult times in life

5. Family and health care guidelines for self-care consist of _____.

A. maintaining a calm atmosphere during the day and using restraints

B. giving step-by-step instruction whenever necessary

C. beginning bowel and bladder program late

II Match each medical term in Column A with its explanation in Column B.

Column A	Column B
_____　1. perseveration	a. a drug that reduces excitability and calms a person
_____　2. neuroleptic	b. continuing or repeating one's behaviour

	3. restraint	c. tranquilizer used to treat psychotic conditions
	4. sedative	d. a rule or condition that limits freedom
	5. regression	e. returning to a former state

III Find words or terms in the article to match the following definitions.

1. loss of language ability _____

2. loss of purposeful movement in the absence of motor or sensory impairment _____

3. loss of sensory ability to recognize objects _____

4. the ability to hide severe deficits_____

IV Critical thinking.

According to the case at the beginning of this unit, what are the nursing diagnoses and the nursing interventions for the patient?

1. Nursing diagnoses

• Impaired verbal communication related to the memory loss and the language disorder

• Altered nutrition: less than the body requirements related to dysphagia and in difficulty in handling complex tasks

• Risk of the injury related to unsteady gait, reduced memory and judgement, and fatigue

2. Nursing interventions

In the early stage of illness, it's necessary to avoid fatigue and keep the patient active. Provide simple explanations and allow sufficient time for verbalization to reduce frustration in communication. Monitoring weight, dysphagia, and diet helps meet nutritional needs. The patient should be monitored carefully, especially at night, when falling and injuring become easier. Teaching the family such basics as bathing, feeding and toileting may be helpful.

Part 4 Supplementary Reading

🎧 Electroconvulsive Therapy

Electroconvulsive therapy (ECT), formerly known as electroshock therapy, and often referred to as shock treatment, is a psychiatric treatment in which seizures are electrically induced in patients to provide relief from mental disorders. The ECT procedure was first conducted in 1938 and is the only currently used form of shock therapy in psychiatry. ECT is often used with informed consent as a last line of intervention for major depressive disorder, mania, and catatonia.

ECT is usually administered three times a week, on alternate days, over a course of two to four weeks. A usual course of ECT involves multiple administrations, typically given two or three times per week until the patient is no longer suffering symptoms. ECT is administered under anaesthetic with a muscle relaxant. Electroconvulsive therapy can differ in its application in three ways: electrode placement, frequency of treatments, and the electrical waveform of the stimulus. These three forms of application have significant differences in both adverse side effects and symptom remission.

The placement of electrodes, as well as the dose and duration of the stimulation is determined on a per-patient basis. Placement can be bilateral, in which the electric current is passed across the whole brain, or unilateral, in which the current is passed across one hemisphere of the brain.

In unilateral ECT, both electrodes are placed on the same side of the patient's head. Unilateral ECT may be used first to minimize side effects such as memory loss. In bilateral ECT, the two electrodes are placed on both sides of the head. Invariably, the bitemporal placement is used, whereby the electrodes are placed on the temples. Uncommonly, the bifrontal placement is used; this involves positioning the electrodes on the patient's forehead, roughly above each eye. Unilateral ECT is thought to cause fewer cognitive effects than bilateral treatment, but is less effective unless administered at higher doses. Bilateral placement seems to have greater efficacy than unilateral, but also carries greater risk of memory loss.

The patient's EEG, ECG, and blood oxygen levels are monitored during the treatment. After the treatment, drug therapy is usually continued, and some patients receive maintenance ECT.

A round of ECT is effective for about 50% of the people with treatment-resistant major depressive disorder, whether it is unipolar or bipolar. The follow-up treatment is still poorly studied, but about half of the people who respond relapse within 12 months. Aside from effects in the brain, the general physical risks of ECT are similar to those of brief general anaesthesia. Immediately following treatment, the most common adverse effects are confusion and memory loss. ECT is considered one of the least harmful treatment options available for severely depressed pregnant women.

Exercise

Choose the best answer to each question based on the text.

1. Which of the following statements is true according to the first paragraph? _____.

   A. ECT provides relief for patients from physical disorders

   B. ECT doesn't require the informed consent of the patient

   C. ECT is the only currently used form of shock therapy in psychiatry

2. ECT differs in its application in the following ways except in the _____.

   A. adverse side effects

   B. frequency of treatments

   C. electrical waveform of the stimulus

3. The placement of electrodes can be _____.

   A. unilateral, in which the electric current is passed across the whole brain

   B. determined on a per-patient basis

   C. bilateral, in which the current is passed across one hemisphere of the brain

4. Bilateral ECT _____.

   A. minimizes side effects such as memory loss

   B. carries greater risk of memory loss

   C. involves positioning the electrodes on the same side of the patient's head

5. Which of the following statements is NOT true according to the last paragraph? _____.

   A. ECT is not suitable for a severely depressed pregnant woman

   B. ECT is effective for about 50% of the people with unipolar and bipolar treatment-resistant depressive disorders

   C. The general physical risks of ECT are similar to those of brief general anaesthesia

Part 5 Medical Word Elements

1. hemi-; semi-	半
hemianopia / ˌhemɪəˈnəʊpɪə /	偏盲
semisupination / ˌsemɪˌsjupɪˈneɪʃn /	半仰卧位
2. hyster(o)-	子宫，癔症
hysteria / hɪˈstɪərɪə /	癔症，歇斯底里
hysteromyoma / ˌhɪstərəmaɪˈəʊmə /	子宫肌瘤
3. -phobia	恐怖
agoraphobia / ˌægərəˈfəʊbɪə /	广场恐怖症
acrophobia / ˌækrəʊˈfəʊbɪə /	恐高症
4. psych(o)-	精神（的），心理（的）
psychosis / saɪˈkəʊsɪs /	精神病，精神错乱
psychotherapy / ˌsaɪkəʊˈθerəpi /	精神疗法
5. schiz(o)-	分裂
schizoaffective / ˌskɪzəʊəˈfektɪv /	情感性分裂的
schizophrenia / ˌskɪzəʊˈfriːnɪə /	精神分裂症
6. -mania	狂，癖
megalomania / ˌmegələʊˈmeɪnɪə /	夸大狂
necromania / nekrəʊˈmeɪnɪə /	恋尸癖
7. -ia	情况，状况
neurasthenia / ˌnjʊərəsˈθiːnɪə /	神经衰弱症
mania / ˈmeɪnɪə /	躁狂症

8. -ism 状态，情况

　　alcoholism / ˈælkəhɒlɪzəm / 酒精中毒

　　paralogism / pəˈrælədʒɪzəm / 谬论，悖理

9. par(a)- 不正常

　　paramnesia / ˌpəræmˈnɪzɪə / 记忆错误

　　paranoid / ˈpærənɔɪd / 患妄想狂的人，偏执狂患者

（罗晓冰　赵　静）

References

阿鲁姆，麦加尔，2010. 护理英语 1. 北京：中国青年出版社

陈沁，王炎峰，2016. 医学专业英语. 第 3 版. 北京：科学出版社

格伦迪宁，霍华德，2010. 剑桥医学英语. 北京：人民邮电出版社

关青，2013. 护理专业英语. 南京：江苏科学技术出版社

黄刚娅，包茹，2013. 护理英语. 成都：西南交通大学出版社

姜安丽，冯先琼，李小寒，等，2005. 护理学基础. 北京：人民卫生出版社

江晓东，2008. 实用护理英语. 重庆：重庆大学出版社

李小寒，尚少梅，2017. 基础护理学. 第 6 版. 北京：人民卫生出版社

孙雪梅，王月贞，2017. 新核心高职行业英语：医护英语. 上海：上海交通大学出版社

吴姣鱼，张亚妮，2013. 护理学基础. 第 2 版. 北京：科学出版社

BALL J, BINDLER R, 1995. Pediatric Nursing: Caring for Children. Norwalk Connecticut: Appleton & Lang

BEARE P G, MYERS J L, 1998. Adult Health Nursing. 3rd edition. St. Louis: Mosby

BILLINGS D M, 2002. Review for NCLEX-RN. 7th edition. Philadelphia: Lippincott

BRAUNWALD E, 1997. Heart Disease: A Textbook of Cardiovascular Medicine. 5th Edition. Philadelphia: Saunders

CRAVEN R F, HIRNLE C J, 2003. Fundamentals of Nursing Human Health and Function. 4th edition. Philadelphia: Lippincott

DECRAMER M, JANSSENS W, MIRAVITLLES M, 2012. Chronic obstructive pulmonary disease. Lancet, 379 (9823)

GRUENDEMANN B J, FERNSEBNER B, 1995. Comprehensive Perioperative Volume 2 Practice Nursing. London: Jones and Bartlett

HALTER M J, 2017. Varcarolis' Foundations of Psychiatric Mental Health Nursing. 8th Edition. Philadelphia: Saunders

JARVIS C, 2000. Physical Examination and Health Assessment. 3rd edition. Philadelphia: Saunders

LEWIS S L, BUCHER L, 2016. Medical-Surgical Nursing: Assessment and Management of Clinical Problems. 10th edition. St. Louis: Mosby

LOPEZ A D, SHIBUYA K, RAO C, et al, 2006. Chronic obstructive pulmonary disease: current burden and future projections. Eur Respir J, 27(2)

LOWDERMILK D L, PERRY S E, BOBAK I M, 1997. Maternity & Women's Health Care. 6th edition. St. Louis: Mosby

PERRY A G, POTTER P A, 1994. Clinical Nursing Skills & Techniques. 3rd edition. St. Louis: Mosby

PIROZZI C, SCHOLAND M B, 2012. Smoking cessation and environmental hygiene. Medical Clinics of North America, 96 (4)

RABE K F, HURD S, ANZUETO A, et al, 2007. Global strategy for the diagnosis, management, and prevention of chronic obstructive pulmonary disease: GOLD executive summary. American Journal of Respiratory and Critical Care Medicine, 176 (6)

SEVO M D, 2014. Pediatric Nursing. Philadelphia: F. A. Davis

SMITH S F, DUELL D J, 1992. Clinical Nursing Skills. 3rd edition. Norwalk, Connecticut: Appleton & Lange

SWEARINGEN P L, 1991. Photo Atlas of Nursing Procedures. 2nd edition. Redwood City: Wesley

TAYLOR C, LILLIS C, LEMONE P, 1997. Fundamentals of Nursing: The Art & Science of Nursing Care. Philadelphia: Lippincott

TAYLOR C, LILLIS C, LEMONE P, 2010. Fundamentals of Nursing: The Art & Science of Nursing Care. 3rd edition. Philadelphia: Lippincott

TRESELER K M, 1995. Clinical Laboratory and Diagnostic Tests: Significance and Nursing Implications. 3rd edition. Norwalk, Connecticut: Appleton & Lange

WICKER P, NEILL J O, 2010. Caring for the Perioperative Patient. 2nd edition. Blackwell: Wiley

Basic Requirements of Teaching

  《护理英语阅读分册》依据护理岗位需要组织教材内容，内容编排以医院真实场景为主线，以临床护理工作为框架，以临床病例为导向，涉及基础护理、内科护理、外科护理、妇科护理、产科护理、儿科护理、精神护理等护理专业理论及技能等内容，还涉及医学影像技术、检验技术、用药护理、人际沟通技巧等相关知识，适合已具备一定公共英语基础的高职高专涉外护理专业、护理专业及相关专业学生使用，亦可作为临床护理人员及拟出国工作的护理人员的参考读物。

  各院校可根据实际情况选择学习，建议安排 54~72 学时。

学时分配建议（72 学时）

单元	教学内容	学时数		
		理论	实践	合计
Unit 1	Patient Admission	3	1	4
Unit 2	Patient Discharge	3	1	4
Unit 3	Medication Administration	3	1	4
Unit 4	Wound Care	3	1	4
Unit 5	Medical Specimen	3	1	4
Unit 6	Medical Imaging	3	1	4
Unit 7	Caring for a Preoperative Patient	3	1	4
Unit 8	Caring for a Postoperative Patient	3	1	4
Unit 9	Caring for a Patient with Diabetes	3	1	4
Unit 10	Caring for a Patient with Heart Disease	3	1	4
Unit 11	Caring for a Patient with Hepatitis	3	1	4
Unit 12	Caring for a Child with Pneumonia	3	1	4
Unit 13	Caring for a Patient with Diarrhea	3	1	4
Unit 14	Caring for a Patient with Chronic Obstructive Pulmonary Disease (COPD)	3	1	4
Unit 15	Caring for a Patient with Hip Replacement	3	1	4
Unit 16	Caring for a Pregnant Woman	3	1	4
Unit 17	Caring for a Patient with Stroke	3	1	4
Unit 18	Caring for a Patient with Alzheimer's Disease	3	1	4
总计		54	18	72

Keys to Exercises

Unit 1

Part 1

I. 1. B   2. B   3. C   4. A   5. B

Part 2

I. 1. A   2. B   3. A   4. C   5. B

II. 1. E   2. A   3. B   4. F   5. G   6. C   7. D

Part 3

I. 1. B   2. C   3. C   4. B   5. C

II. 1. e   2. c   3. b   4. d   5. a

III. 1. auscultation   2. tachycardia   3. thermometer   4. sphygmomanometer

Part 4

1. A   2. C   3. A   4. A   5. C

Unit 2

Part 1

I. 1. B   2. A   3. B   4. A   5. C

Part 2

I. 1. A   2. B   3. A   4. B   5. C

II. 1. C   2. F   3. A   4. D   5. E   6. B   7. G

Part 3

I. 1. C   2. C   3. A   4. B   5. A

II. 1. e   2. c   3. d   4. a   5. b

III. 1. caregiver   2. complication   3. intervention   4. treatment

Part 4

1. B   2. B   3. A   4. B   5. B

Unit 3

Part 1

I. 1. A   2. B   3. B   4. C   5. A

Part 2

I. 1. C   2. A   3. B   4. B   5. C

II. 1. D   2. A   3. G   4. E   5. B   6. C   7. F   8. H

Part 3

I. 1. C   2. C   3. B   4. A   5. A

II. 1. c   2. a   3. b   4. e   5. d

III. 1. laxative   2. nebulizer   3. nasogastric   4. parenteral

Part 4

1. A   2. A   3. C   4. A   5. B

Unit 4

Part 1

I. 1. A   2. B   3. A   4. A   5. C

Part 2

I. 1. C   2. C   3. C   4. B   5. C

II. 1. C   2. A   3. D   4. B   5. E   6. F

Part 3

I. 1. B   2. A   3. A   4. C   5. C

II. 1. b   2. c   3. e   4. d   5. a

III. 1. debridement   2. contaminated wound   3. inflammation   4. autolytic

Part 4

1. A   2. A   3. B   4. C   5. B

Unit 5

Part 1

I. 1. A   2. B   3. C   4. B   5. B

Part 2

I. 1. B   2. C   3. B   4. A   5. C

II. 1. E   2. B   3. D   4. G   5. A   6. F   7. C

Part 3

I. 1. C   2. A   3. A   4. B   5. A

II. 1. c   2. a   3. d   4. e   5. b

III. 1. pathologist   2. venipuncture   3. urinalysis   4. sputum

Part 4

1. A   2. C   3. B   4. A   5. B

Unit 6

Part 1

I. 1. B   2. A   3. C   4. A   5. B

Part 2

I. 1. A   2. B   3. B   4. C   5. B

II. 1. E   2. B   3. C   4. G   5. D   6. A   7. F

Part 3

I. 1. A   2. B   3. C   4. A   5. B

II. 1. e   2. c   3. b   4. d   5. a

III. 1. ultrasonography   2. radiologist   3. obstetrician   4. intestine

Part 4

1. C   2. A   3. C   4. C   5. B

Unit 7

Part 1

I. 1. A   2. B   3. B   4. C   5. B

Part 2

I. 1. C   2. C   3. A   4. C   5. B

II. 1. C   2. G   3. A   4. B   5. E   6. F   7. D

Part 3

I. 1. C   2. A   3. C   4. B   5. A

II. 1. c   2. a   3. b   4. e   5. d

III. 1. deep-breathing   2. communication   3. cross-match   4. assessment

Part 4

1. C   2. B   3. A   4. A   5. A

Unit 8

Part 1

I. 1. C   2. B   3. B   4. A   5. B

Part 2

I. 1. C   2. A   3. C   4. B   5. A

II. 1. B   2. F   3. A   4. E   5. D   6. C   7. G

Part 3

I. 1. A   2. C   3. C   4. B   5. C

II. 1. b   2. a   3. c   4. d   5. e

III. 1. nausea   2. lumen   3. swelling   4. appendix

Part 4

1. A   2. B   3. B   4. B   5. B

Unit 9

Part 1

I. 1. A   2. B   3. B   4. C   5. B

Part 2

I. 1. A   2. B   3. C   4. C   5. B

II. 1. B   2. C   3. D   4. F   5. G   6. A   7. E

Part 3

I. 1. B   2. C   3. B   4. C   5. B

II. 1. c   2. a   3. b   4. e   5. d

III. 1. carbohydrates   2. protein   3. pancreas   4. retinopathy

Part 4

1. C   2. A   3. C   4. B   5. C

Unit 10

Part 1

I. 1. A   2. B   3. A   4. B   5. C

Part 2

I. 1. B   2. C   3. A   4. C   5. B

II. 1. D   2. B   3. G   4. E   5. F   6. C   7. A

Part 3

I. 1. C   2. C   3. B   4. A   5. A

II. 1. e   2. c   3. a   4. b   5. d

III. 1. heart failure   2. left ventricle   3. bypass surgery   4. pacemaker

Part 4

1. A   2. B   3. A   4. B   5. C

Unit 11

Part 1

I. 1. A   2. B   3. B   4. A   5. A

Part 2

I. 1. B   2. A   3. B   4. C   5. C

II. 1. D   2. F   3. A   4. E   5. B   6. G   7. H   8. C

Part 3

I. 1. B   2. C   3. A   4. B   5. C

II. 1. d   2. a   3. e   4. c   5. b

III. 1. malaise   2. sedative   3. concentration   4. autoimmune   5. lethargy

Part 4

1. C   2. C   3. C   4. C   5. A

Unit 12

Part 1

I. 1. A   2. B   3. A   4. B   5. C

Part 2

I. 1. C   2. A   3. C   4. B   5. A

II. 1. C   2. F   3. D   4. A   5. G   6. E   7. B   8. H

Part 3

I. 1. C   2. A   3. B   4. C   5. A

II. 1. c   2. a   3. b   4. e   5. d

III. 1. tachypnoea   2. antipyretic   3. pneumococcus   4. antibiotics

Part 4

1. C   2. A   3. C   4. A   5. B

Unit 13

Part 1

I. 1. A   2. B   3. A   4. B   5. A

Part 2

I. 1. C   2. B   3. A   4. B   5. A

II. 1. E   2. H   3. G   4. F   5. A   6. D   7. C   8. B

Part 3

I. 1. C   2. C   3. B   4. C   5. B

II. 1. c   2. a   3. d   4. b   5. e

III. 1. diarrhoea   2. cholera   3. hyperthyroidism   4. colitis

Part 4

1. A   2. B   3. A   4. C   5. B

Unit 14

Part 1

I. 1. A   2. B   3. A   4. B   5. A

Part 2

I. 1. C   2. B   3. A   4. B   5. C

II. 1. F   2. D   3. E   4. C   5. B   6. A

Part 3

I. 1. B   2. C   3. A   4. C   5. B

II. 1. e   2. a   3. d   4. b   5. c

III. 1. emphysema   2. chronic bronchitis   3. bronchodilator   4. inhalation

Part 4

I. 1. C   2. C   3. A   4. A   5. B

Unit 15

Part 1

I. 1. B   2. A   3. B   4. C   5. B

Part 2

I. 1. C   2. A   3. B   4. C   5. B

II. 1. D   2. A   3. F   4. C   5. B   6. E   7. G

Part 3

I. 1. C   2. A   3. B   4. C   5. C

II. 1. b   2. c   3. e   4. a   5. d

III. 1. hip replacement   2. total hip replacement / total hip arthroplasty

3. hemi hip replacement / hemiarthroplasty

4. general anaesthesia   5. blood transfusion

Part 4

1. C   2. C   3. C   4. A   5. A

Unit 16

Part 1

I. 1. B   2. B   3. A   4. C   5. B

Part 2

I. 1. C   2. B   3. C   4. C   5. A

II. 1. C   2. A   3. F   4. D   5. B   6. E

Part 3

I. 1. A   2. B   3. C   4. B   5. B

II. 1. b   2. c   3. d   4. a   5. e

III. 1. PIH   2. fluid retention   3. swelling

 4. hypertension   5. delivery

Part 4

1. B   2. C   3. A   4. C   5. A

Unit 17

Part 1

I. 1. A   2. B   3. B   4. A   5. C

Part 2

I. 1. A   2. C   3. A   4. A   5. B

II. 1. F   2. A   3. C   4. B   5. G   6. E   7. D

Part 3

I. 1. C   2. C   3. A   4. B   5. C

II. 1. c   2. a   3. b   4. e   5. d

III. 1. dysarthria   2. congenital   3. thrombosis   4. edema

Part 4

1. A   2. A   3. B   4. C   5. C

Unit 18

Part 1

I. 1. B   2. B   3. A   4. A   5. A

Part 2

I. 1. C   2. A   3. C   4. B   5. C

II. 1. B   2. C   3. D   4. A

Part 3

I. 1. B   2. C   3. A   4. C   5. B

II. 1. b   2. c   3. d   4. a   5. e

III. 1. aphasia   2. apraxia   3. agnosia   4. denial

Part 4

1. B   2. A   3. B   4. B   5. A